Cotton and Williams'
Practical Gastrointestinal Endoscopy
The Fundamentals

Cotton and Williams' Practical Gastrointestinal Endoscopy

The Fundamentals

Adam Haycock MBBS BSc(hons) MRCP MD FHEA

Consultant Physician and Gastroenterologist
Honorary Senior Lecturer
Imperial College; *and*
Endoscopy Training Lead
Wolfson Unit for Endoscopy
St Mark's Hospital for Colorectal and Intestinal Disorders
London, UK

Jonathan Cohen MD FASGE FACG

Clinical Professor of Medicine
Division of Gastroenterology
New York University School of Medicine
New York, USA

Brian P Saunders MD FRCP

Consultant Gastroenterologist
St Mark's Hospital for Colorectal and Intestinal Disorders; *and*
Adjunct Professor of Endoscopy
Imperial College
London, UK

Peter B Cotton MD FRCP FRCS

Professor of Medicine
Digestive Disease Center
Medical University of South Carolina
Charleston, South Carolina, USA

Christopher B Williams BM FRCP FRCS

Honorary Physician
Wolfson Unit for Endoscopy
St Mark's Hospital for Colorectal and Intestinal Disorders
London, UK

Videos supplied by Stephen Preston
Multimedia Consultant
St Mark's Hospital for Colorectal and Intestinal Disorders
London, UK

WILEY Blackwell

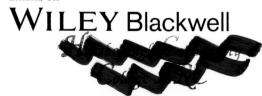

This edition first published 2014© 1980, 1982, 1990, 1996, 2003 by Blackwell Publishing Ltd, 2008 by Peter B Cotton, Christopher B Williams, Robert H Hawes and Brian P Saunders, 2014 by John Wiley & Sons, Ltd.

Registered office: John Wiley & Sons, Ltd, The Atrium, Southern Gate, Chichester, West Sussex, PO19 8SQ, UK

Editorial offices: 9600 Garsington Road, Oxford, OX4 2DQ, UK
The Atrium, Southern Gate, Chichester, West Sussex, PO19 8SQ, UK
111 River Street, Hoboken, NJ 07030-5774, USA

For details of our global editorial offices, for customer services and for information about how to apply for permission to reuse the copyright material in this book please see our website at www.wiley.com/wiley-blackwell

Library of Congress Cataloging-in-Publication Data

Haycock, Adam, author.
  Cotton and Williams' practical gastrointestinal endoscopy : the fundamentals / Adam Haycock, Jonathan Cohen, Brian P. Saunders, Peter B. Cotton, Christopher B. Williams ; videos supplied by Stephen Preston.—7th edition.
      p. ; cm.
  Practical gastrointestinal endoscopy
  Preceded by: Practical gastrointestinal endoscopy / Peter B. Cotton . . . [et al.]. 6th ed. 2008.
  Includes bibliographical references.
    ISBN 978-1-118-40646-5 (cloth)
  I. Cohen, Jonathan, 1964– author. II. Saunders, Brian P., author. III. Cotton, Peter B., author. IV. Williams, Christopher B. (Christopher Beverley), author. V. Title. VI. Title: Practical gastrointestinal endoscopy.
  [DNLM: 1. Gastrointestinal Diseases–diagnosis. 2. Endoscopy–methods. 3. Gastrointestinal Diseases–surgery. WI 141]
  RC804.G3
  616.3'307545–dc23
                            2013041985

A catalogue record for this book is available from the British Library.

Wiley also publishes its books in a variety of electronic formats. Some content that appears in print may not be available in electronic books.

Cover image: background image from the authors, inset images by David Gardner
Cover design by Sarah Dickinson

Set in 8.5/11 pt Meridien by Toppan Best-set Premedia Limited
Printed and bound in Singapore by Markono Print Media Pte Ltd

02 2015

Contents

List of Video Clips

Preface to the Seventh Edition

Gastrointestinal endoscopy continues to evolve and has seen a steady increase in demand, complexity, and innovation in what it is possible to do with an endoscope. It is now the undoubted investigation of choice for the GI tract, although there is no room for complacency. Parallel improvements in imaging capabilities such as MRCP and CT colonography are now impacting on the "diagnostic" endoscopy workload, and much of the current emphasis is on advancing endoluminal, transluminal, and hybrid therapeutic techniques.

The ongoing adoption of national bowel cancer screening programs has driven up standards for endoscopists across the board. Increasing recognition of the importance of identifying even small, subtle premalignant dysplastic lesions and the ability to provide complex therapeutic intervention in both the upper and lower GI tract has made the learning process even more lengthy and difficult for those new to the field. Accordingly, the "fundamentals" no longer refers solely to basic or simple procedures, if indeed it ever did. In this era of increasing complexity of endoscopy and increasing attention to quality performance, the fundamental skills that constitute the foundation of all endoscopic practice have never been more important to master.

In line with the last edition, we have limited this book to the most common diagnostic and therapeutic "upper" and "lower" GI procedures, reserving more advanced techniques such as ERCP and EUS for others to cover. What is new to this edition is acknowledgement of the enormous impact of the Internet and electronic "e-learning." This edition is supported by a selection of online multimedia images and clips, which are signposted in the text and referenced at the end of each chapter. To allow for greater use of mobile platforms, each chapter has been reconfigured into a more easily digestible "bite-sized" chunk with its own key learning points and searchable keywords. Multiple-choice questions (MCQs) are also available online to allow self-assessment and consolidate learning.

We also formally acknowledge with this edition what has been common parlance for years—that this book is "Cotton and Williams'" fundamentals of gastrointestinal endoscopy, sharing personal opinions, tips, and tricks gained over many years. Although this is the last edition in which these two pioneering authors will actively participate, this textbook will remain a practical guide squarely based on their practice and principles. It has been our privilege to work with them to produce this edition, and we are honored to have been asked to sustain this important effort in the future.

Practical Gastrointestinal Endoscopy: The Fundamentals aims to complement rather than replace more evidence-based recommendations and guidelines produced by national societies. It remains focused on helping those in the first few years of experience to move more quickly up the learning curve toward competency. We hope that it will inspire trainees to attain the levels of excellence represented by those individuals from whom the book takes its name.

Adam Haycock
Jonathan Cohen
Brian P Saunders

Preface to the First Edition

This book is concerned with endoscopic techniques and says little about their clinical relevance. It does so unashamedly because no comparable manual was available at the time of its conception and because the explosive growth of endoscopy has far outstripped facilities for individual training in endoscopic technique. For the same reason we have made no mention of rigid endoscopes (oesophagoscopes, sigmoidoscopes and laparoscopes) which rightly remain popular tools in gastroenterology, nor have we discussed the great potential of the flexible endoscope in gastrointestinal research.

Our concentration on techniques should not be taken to denote a lack of interest in results and real indications. As gastroenterologists we believe that procedures can only be useful if they improve our clinical management; clever techniques are not indicated simply because they are possible, and some endoscopic procedures will become obsolete with improvements in less invasive methods. Indeed we are moving into a self-critical phase in which the main interest in gastrointestinal endoscopy is in the assessment of its real role and cost-effectiveness.

Gastrointestinal endoscopy should be only one of the tools of specialists trained in gastrointestinal disease—whether they are primarily physicians, surgeons or radiologists. Only with broad training and knowledge is it possible to place obscure endoscopic findings in their relevant clinical perspective, to make realistic judgements in the selection of complex investigations from different disciplines, and to balance the benefits and risks of new therapeutic applications. Some specialists will become more expert and committed than others, but we do not favour the widespread development of pure endoscopists or of endoscopy as a subspecialty.

Skilful endoscopy can often provide a definitive diagnosis and lead quickly to correct management, which may save patients from months or years of unnecessary illness or anxiety. We hope that this little book may help to make that process easier and safer.

April 1979
P.B.C., C.B.W.

Acknowledgments

The authors are grateful to the dedicated collaborators who have embellished or enabled the production of this book.

The skills of Steve Preston (steveprestonmultimedia@gmail.com) produced the web videos and imagery. The artistry and great patience of David Gardner (davidgardner@cytanet.com.cy) has allowed upgrading of the drawings and figures in this edition and several previous ones. At Wiley publishers, the guidance of Oliver Walter, backed by Rebecca Huxley's formidable editorial talents, has made the production process almost enjoyable.

The authors also wish to register indebtedness to their respective life-partners (Cori, Sarah, Annie, Marion and Christina) for their unending support—despite intrusions into personal and family time.

About the Companion Website

This book is accompanied by a website:

www.wiley.com/go/cottonwilliams/practicalgastroenterology

The website includes:

- 37 videos showing procedures described in the book
- All videos are referenced in the text where you see this logo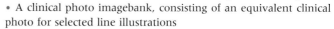
- A clinical photo imagebank, consisting of an equivalent clinical photo for selected line illustrations
- An interactive "check your understanding" question bank (MCQs) to test main learning points in each chapter

CHAPTER 1

The Endoscopy Unit, Staff, and Management

Most endoscopists, and especially beginners, focus on the individual procedures and have little appreciation of the extensive infrastructure that is now necessary for efficient and safe activity. From humble beginnings in adapted single rooms, most of us are lucky enough now to work in large units with multiple procedure rooms full of complex electronic equipment, with additional space dedicated to preparation, recovery, and reporting.

Endoscopy is a team activity, requiring the collaborative talents of many people with different backgrounds and training. It is difficult to overstate the importance of appropriate facilities and adequate professional support staff, to maintain patient comfort and safety, and to optimize clinical outcomes.

Endoscopy procedures can be performed almost anywhere when necessary (e.g. in an intensive care unit), but the vast majority take place in purpose-designed "endoscopy units."

Endoscopy units

Details of endoscopy unit design are beyond the scope of this book, but certain principles should be stated.

There are two types of unit. Private clinics (called ambulatory surgical centers in the USA) deal mainly with healthy (or relatively healthy) outpatients, and should resemble cheerful modern dental suites. Hospital units have to provide a safe environment for managing sick inpatients, and also more complex procedures with a therapeutic focus, such as endoscopic retrograde cholangiopancreatography (ERCP). The more sophisticated units resemble operating suites. Units that serve both functions should be designed to separate the patient flows as far as possible.

The modern unit has areas designed for many different functions. Like a hotel or an airport (or a Victorian household), the endoscopy unit should have a smart public face ("upstairs"), and a more functional back hall ("downstairs"). From the patient's perspective, the suite consists of areas devoted to reception, preparation, procedure, recovery, and discharge. Supporting these activities are many other "back hall" functions, which include scheduling, cleaning, preparation, maintenance and storage of equipment, reporting and archiving, and staff management.

Cotton and Williams' Practical Gastrointestinal Endoscopy: The Fundamentals, Seventh Edition.
Adam Haycock, Jonathan Cohen, Brian P Saunders, Peter B Cotton, and Christopher B Williams.
© 2014 John Wiley & Sons, Ltd. Published 2014 by John Wiley & Sons, Ltd.
Companion Website: www.wiley.com/go/cottonwilliams/practicalgastroenterology

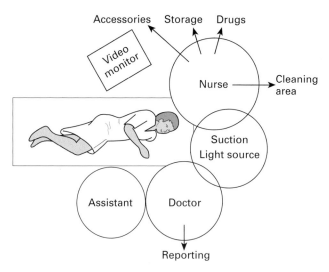

Fig 1.1 Functional planning—spheres of activity.

Procedure rooms

The rooms used for endoscopy procedures should:
- *not be cluttered or intimidating*. Most patients are not sedated when they enter, so it is better for the room to resemble a modern dental office, or kitchen, rather than an operating room.
- *be large enough* to allow a patient stretcher/trolley to be rotated on its axis, and to accommodate all of the equipment and staff (and any emergency team), but also compact enough for efficient function.
- *be laid out with function in mind*, keeping nursing and doctor spheres of activity separate (Fig 1.1), and minimizing exposed trailing electrical cables and pipes (best by ceiling-mounted beams).

Each room should have:
- *piped oxygen and suction* (two lines);
- *lighting planned* to illuminate nursing activities but not dazzle the patient or endoscopist;
- *video monitors placed conveniently* for the endoscopist and assistants, but also allowing the patient to view, if wished;
- *adequate counter space* for accessories, with a large sink or receptacle for dirty equipment;
- *storage space for equipment required on a daily basis*;
- *systems of communication* with the charge nurse desk, and emergency call;
- *disposal systems* for hazardous materials.

Patient preparation and recovery areas

Patients need a private place for initial preparation (undressing, safety checks, intravenous (IV) access), and a similar place in which to recover from any sedation or anesthesia. In some units these functions are separate, but can be combined to maximize flexibility. Many units have simple curtained bays, but rooms with solid side walls and a movable front curtain are preferable. They should be large enough to accommodate at least two people other than the patient on the stretcher, and all of the necessary monitoring equipment.

The "prep-recovery bays" should be adjacent to a central nursing workstation. Like the bridge of a ship, it is where the nurse captain of the day controls and steers the whole operation, and from which recovering patients can be monitored.

All units should have at least one completely private room for sensitive interviews/consultations before and after procedures.

Equipment management and storage

There must be designated areas for endoscope and accessory reprocessing, and storage of medications and all equipment, including an emergency resuscitation cart. Many units also have fully equipped mobile carts to travel to other sites when needed.

Staff

Specially trained endoscopy assistants have many important functions. They:
* *prepare patients* for their procedures, physically and mentally;
* *set up* all necessary equipment;
* *assist* endoscopists during procedures;
* *monitor* patients' safety, sedation, and recovery;
* *clean*, disinfect, and process equipment;
* *maintain quality control*.

Most endoscopy assistants are trained nurses, but technicians and nursing aides also have roles (e.g. in equipment processing). Large units need a variety of other staff, to handle reception, transport, reporting, and equipment management, including informatics.

Members of staff need places to store their clothes and valuables, and a break area for refreshments and meals.

Procedure reports

Usually, two reports are generated for each procedure—one by the nurses and one by the endoscopist.

Nurse's report

The nurse's report usually takes the form of a preprinted "flow sheet," with places to record all of the pre-procedure safety checks, vital signs, use of sedation/analgesia and other medications, monitoring of vital signs and patient responses, equipment and accessory usage, and image documentation. It concludes with a copy of the discharge instructions given to the patient.

Endoscopist's report

In many units, the endoscopist's report is written or dictated in the procedure rooms. In larger ones, there may need to be a separate area designed for that purpose.

The endoscopist's report includes the patient's demographics, reasons for the procedure (indications), specific medical risks and precautions, sedation/analgesia, findings, diagnostic specimens, treatments, conclusions, follow-up plans, and any unplanned events (complications). Endoscopists use many reporting methods—handwritten notes, preprinted forms, free dictation, and computer databases.

The paperless endoscopy unit

Eventually all of the documentation (nursing, administrative, and endoscopic) will be incorporated into a comprehensive electronic management system. Such a system will substantially reduce the paperwork burden, and increase both efficiency and quality control.

Management, behavior, and teamwork

Complex organizations require efficient management and leadership. This works best as a collaborative exercise between the medical director of endoscopy and the chief nurse or endoscopy nurse manager. The biggest units will also have a separate administrator. These individuals must be skilled in handling people (doctors, staff, and patients), complex equipment, and significant financial resources. They must develop and maintain good working relationships with many departments within the hospital (such as radiology, pathology, sterile processing, anesthesia, bioengineering), as well as numerous manufacturers and vendors. They also need to be fully cognizant of all of the many local and national regulations that now impact on endoscopy practice.

The wise endoscopist will embrace the team approach, and realize that maintaining an atmosphere of collegiality and mutual respect is essential for efficiency, job satisfaction, and staff retention, and for optimal patient outcomes.

It is also essential to ensure that the push for efficiency does not drive out humanity. Patients should not be packaged as mere commodities during the endoscopy process. Treating our customers (and those who accompany them) with respect and courtesy is fundamental. Always assume that patients are listening, even if apparently sedated, so never chatter about irrelevances in their presence. Never eat or drink in patient areas. Background music is appreciated by many patients and staff.

Documentation and quality improvement

The agreed policies of the unit (including regulations dictated by the hospital and national organizations) are enshrined in an *Endoscopy Unit Procedure Manual*. This must be easily available, constantly updated, and frequently consulted.

Day-to-day documentation includes details of staff and room usage, disinfection processes, medications, instrument and accessory use and problems, as well as the procedure reports.

A formal quality assessment and improvement process is essential for maximizing the safety and efficiency of endoscopy services. Professional societies have recommended methods and metrics. The American Society for Gastrointestinal Endoscopy (ASGE) has incorporated these into its Endoscopy Unit Recognition Program, and the benefit of concentrating on and documenting quality is well exemplified by the success of the Global Rating Scale project in the UK.

Educational resources

Endoscopy units should offer educational resources for all of its users, including patients, staff, and doctors. Clinical staff need a selection of relevant books, atlases, key reprints, and journals, and publications of professional societies. Increasingly, many of these materials are available online, so that easy Internet access should be available. Many organizations produce useful educational videotapes, CD-ROMs, and DVDs.

Teaching units will need to embrace computer simulators, which are becoming valuable tools for training (and credentialing).

Further reading

Armstrong D, Barkun A, Cotton PB *et al*. Canadian Association of Gastroenterology consensus guidelines on safety and quality indicators in endoscopy. *Can J Gastroenterol* 2012; **26**: 17–31.

ASGE Quality Assurance In Endoscopy Committee, Petersen BT, Chennat J *et al*. Multisociety guideline on reprocessing flexible gastrointestinal endoscopes. *Gastrointest Endosc* 2011; **73**: 1075–84.

Cotton PB. Quality endoscopists and quality endoscopy units. *J Interv Gastroenterol* 2011; **1**: 83–7.

Cotton PB, Bretthauer M. Quality assurance in gastroenterology. *Best Pract Res Clin Gastroenterol* 2011; **25**: 335–6.

Cotton PB, Barkun A, Hawes RH, Ginsberg G (eds) *Efficiency in Endoscopy. Gastrointestinal Endoscopy Clinics of North America*, Vol. **14**(4) (series ed. Lightdale CJ). Philadelphia: WB Saunders, 2004.

Faigel DO, Cotton PB. The London OMED position statement for credentialing and quality assurance in digestive endoscopy. *Endoscopy* 2009; **41**: 1069–74.

Global Rating Scale. (available online at www.globalratingscale.com).

JAG (British Joint Advisory Group on GI Endoscopy). (available online at http://www.thejag.org.uk/AboutUs/DownloadCentre.aspx).

Petersen B, Ott B. Design and management of gastrointestinal endoscopy units. In: *Advanced Digestive Endoscopy e-book/annual: Endoscopic Practice and Safety*. Blackwell Publishing, 2008. (available online at www.gastrohep.com).

Chapter video clip

Video 1.1 The endoscopy unit: a virtual tour

Now check your understanding—go to
www.wiley.com/go/cottonwilliams/practicalgastroenterology

CHAPTER 2

Endoscopic Equipment

Endoscopes

There are many different endoscopes available for various applications, and several manufacturers, but they all have common features. There is a control head with valves (buttons) for air insufflation and suction, a flexible shaft (insertion tube) carrying the light guide and one or more service channels, and a maneuverable bending section at the tip. An umbilical or universal cord (also called "light guide connecting tube") connects the endoscope to the light source and processor, air supply, and suction (Fig 2.1). Illumination is provided from an external high-intensity source through one or more light-carrying fiber bundles.

The image is captured with a charge-coupled device (CCD) chip, transmitted electronically, and displayed on a video monitor. Individual pixels (photo cells) in the CCD chips can respond only to degrees of light and dark. Color appreciation is arranged by two methods. So-called "color CCDs" have their pixels arranged under a series of color filter stripes (Fig 2.2). By contrast, "monochrome CCDs" (or, more correctly, sequential system CCDs) use a rotating color filter wheel to illuminate all of the pixels with primary color strobe-effect lighting (Fig 2.3). This type of chip can be made smaller, or can give higher resolution, but the system is more expensive because of the additional mechanics and image-processing technology.

"Electronic chromoendoscopy" systems are now standard in many endoscopes, allowing enhancement of aspects of the surface of the gastrointestinal mucosa. Narrow band imaging (NBI; Olympus Corporation) uses optical filters to select certain wavelengths of light, which correspond to the peak light absorption of hemoglobin, enhancing the visualization of blood vessels and certain surface structures. The Fuji Intelligent Chromo Endoscopy (FICE; Fujinon Endoscopy) and i-Scan (Pentax Medical) systems take ordinary endoscopic images and digitally process the output to estimate different wavelengths of light, providing a number of different imaging outputs. Autofluorescence imaging can detect endogenous fluorophores, a number of which occur in the gastrointestinal tract. Two systems now also allow magnification of the endoscopic image down to the cellular level: termed confocal microscopy (Pentax Medical, Mauna Kea Technologies). Blue laser

Cotton and Williams' Practical Gastrointestinal Endoscopy: The Fundamentals, Seventh Edition.
Adam Haycock, Jonathan Cohen, Brian P Saunders, Peter B Cotton, and Christopher B Williams.
© 2014 John Wiley & Sons, Ltd. Published 2014 by John Wiley & Sons, Ltd.
Companion Website: www.wiley.com/go/cottonwilliams/practicalgastroenterology

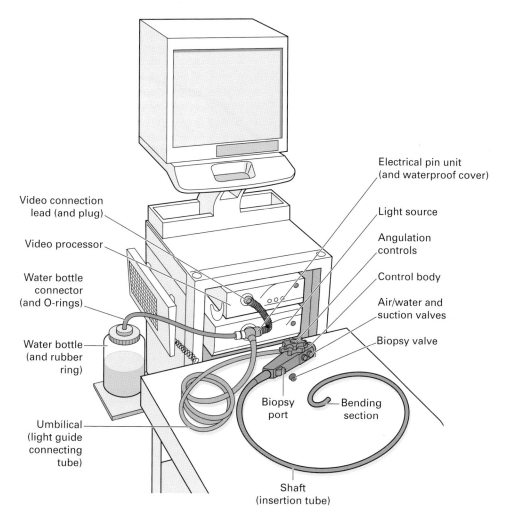

Fig 2.1 Endoscope system.

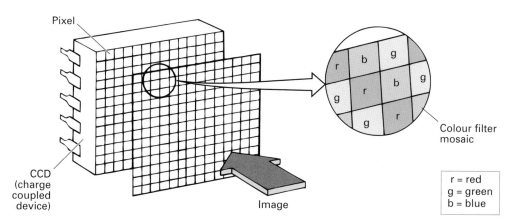

Fig 2.2 Static red, green, and blue filters in the "color" chip.

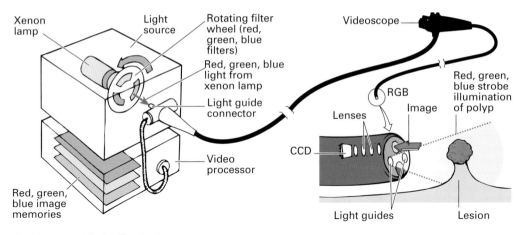

Fig 2.3 Sequential color illumination.

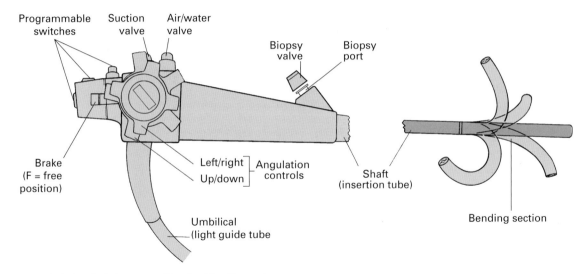

Fig 2.4 Basic design—control head and bending section.

light is focused on the desired tissue after injecting fluorescent materials, which become excited by the laser light and are detected at defined horizontal levels.

Tip control

The distal bending section (10 cm or so) and tip of the endoscope is fully deflectable, usually in both planes, up to 180° or more. Control depends upon pull wires attached at the tip just beneath the outer protective sheath, and passing back through the length of the instrument shaft to the two angulation control wheels (for up/down and right/left movement) on the control head (Fig 2.4). The wheels incorporate a friction braking system, so that the tip can be fixed temporarily in any desired position. The instrument shaft is torque stable, so that rotating movements applied to the head are transmitted to the tip when the shaft is relatively straight.

Insertion tube (shaft)   **Control body**

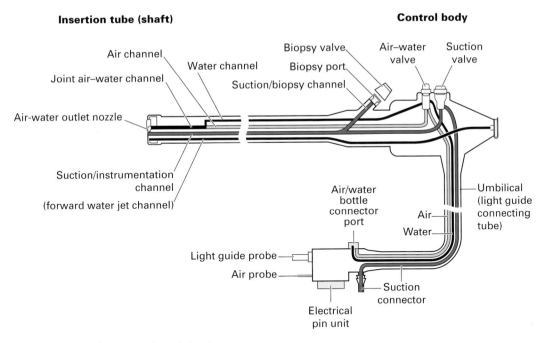

Fig 2.5 The internal anatomy of a typical endoscope.

Instrument channels and valves

The internal anatomy of endoscopes is complex (Fig 2.5). The shaft incorporates a biopsy/suction channel extending from the entry "biopsy port" to the tip of the instrument. The channel is usually about 3 mm in diameter, but varies from 1 to 5 mm depending upon the purpose for which the endoscope was designed (from neonatal examinations to major therapeutic procedures). In some instruments, especially those with lateral-viewing optics, the tip of the channel incorporates a deflectable elevator or bridge (see Fig 2.7), which permits directional control of forceps and other accessories independent of the instrument tip. This elevator is controlled by an additional thumb lever. The biopsy/suction channel is used also for aspirating secretions: an external suction pump is connected to the universal cord near to the light source, and suction is diverted into the instrument channel by pressing the suction valve. Another small channel allows the passage of air to distend the organ being examined. The air is supplied from a pump in the light source and is controlled by another valve. For colonoscopy, the air insufflation system can be modified to CO_2 rather than room air and has been shown to lessen abdominal distension and pain after colonoscopy. The air system also pressurizes the water bottle, so that a jet of water can be squirted across the distal lens to clean it.

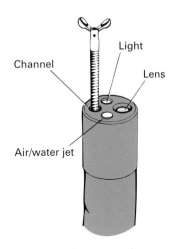

Fig 2.6 The tip of a forward-viewing endoscope.

Different instruments

The endoscopy unit must have a selection of endoscopes for specific applications. These may differ in length, size, stiffness, channel size and number, sophistication, and distal lens orientation. Most

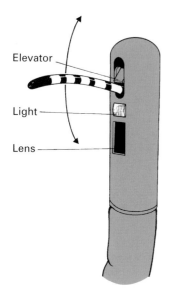

Elevator

Light

Lens

Fig 2.7 A side-viewer with a deflectable elevator.

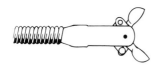

Fig 2.8 Biopsy cups open.

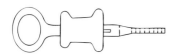

Fig 2.9 Control handle for forceps.

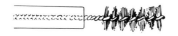

Fig 2.10 Cytology brush with outer sleeve.

endoscopies are performed with instruments providing *direct forward vision*, via a wide-angle lens (up to 130°) (Fig 2.6). However, there are circumstances in which it is preferable to view *laterally*, particularly for endoscopic retrograde cholangiopancreatography (ERCP) (Fig 2.7).

The overall diameter of an endoscope is a compromise between engineering ideals and patient tolerance. The shaft must contain and protect many bundles, wires, and tubes, all of which are stronger and more efficient when larger (Fig 2.5). A colonoscope can reasonably approach 15 m in diameter, but this size is acceptable in the upper gut only for specialized therapeutic instruments.

Routine upper endoscopy is mostly performed with instruments of 8–11 mm diameter. Smaller endoscopes are available; they are better tolerated by all patients and have specific application in children. Some can be passed through the nose rather than the mouth. However, smaller instruments inevitably involve some compromise in durability, image quality, maneuverability, biopsy size, and therapeutic potential.

Several companies now produce a full range of endoscopes at comparable prices. However, light sources and processors produced by different companies are not interchangeable, so that most endoscopy units concentrate for convenience on equipment from a single manufacturer. Endoscopes are delicate, and some breakages are inevitable. Careful maintenance and close communication, repair, and back-up arrangements with an efficient company are necessary to maintain an endoscopy service. The quality of that support is often a crucial factor affecting the choice of company.

Endoscopic accessories

Many devices can be passed through the endoscope biopsy/suction channel for diagnostic and therapeutic purposes.
• *Biopsy forceps* consist of a pair of sharpened cups (Fig 2.8), a spiral metal cable, a pull wire, and a control handle (Fig 2.9). Their maximum diameter is limited by the size of the channel, and the length of the cups by the radius of curvature through which they must pass in the instrument tip. When taking biopsy specimens from a lesion that can only be approached tangentially (e.g. the wall of the esophagus), forceps with a central spike may be helpful; however, these do present a significant puncture hazard for staff.
• *Cytology brushes* have a covering plastic sleeve to protect the specimen during withdrawal (Fig 2.10).
• *Flexible needles* are used for injections and for sampling fluids and cells.
• *Fluid-flushing devices*. Most instruments have a flushing jet channel to keep the lens clean. Fluids can also be forcibly flushed through the instrumentation channel with a large syringe or a pulsatile electric pump, with a suitable nozzle inserted into the biopsy port. For more precise aiming, a washing catheter can be passed down the channel to clean specific areas of interest, or to highlight mucosal detail by "dye spraying" (using a nozzle-tipped catheter).

Ancillary equipment

• *Suction traps* (fitted temporarily into the suction line) can be used to take samples of intestinal secretions and bile for microbiology, chemistry, and cytology (Fig 2.11; see also Fig 7.27).

• *Biteguards* are used to protect the patient's teeth and the endoscope. Some guards have straps, to keep them in place, and oxygen ports.

• *Overtubes* are flexible plastic sleeves that cover the endoscope shaft and act as a conduit for repeated intubations, or to facilitate therapeutic procedures such as the extraction of a foreign body and hemostasis (Fig 2.12).

• *Caps* of various shapes can be attached to the tip of the endoscope to facilitate various procedures, such as banding and mucosal resection, dissection, etc.

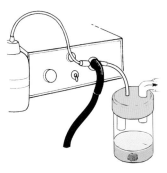

Fig 2.11 A suction trap to collect fluid specimens.

• *Stretchers/trolleys*. Endoscopy is normally performed on a standard transportation stretcher. This should have side rails, and preferably allow height adjustment. The ability to tilt the stretcher head down may be helpful in emergencies.

• *Image documentation*. Videoscopes capture images digitally, which can then be enhanced, stored, transmitted, and printed. Video sequences can be recorded on tape or digitally.

• *Sedation and monitoring*. All patients require regular monitoring during an endoscopy with pulse oximetry as a minimum. Many units also have the facility for continuous blood pressure monitoring and electrocardiography, particularly for deeply sedated patients. Appropriate resuscitation equipment must be available, including oral airways, oxygen delivery systems, and wall suction.

Electrosurgical units

Any electrosurgical unit can be used for endoscopic therapy if necessary, but purpose-built isolated-circuit and "intelligent" units have major advantages in safety and ease of use. Units should have test circuitry and an automatic warning system or cut-out in case a connection is faulty or the patient plate is not in contact. Most units have separate "cut" and "coagulate" circuits, which can often be blended to choice. For flexible endoscopy, low-power settings are used (typically 15–50 W). However, an "auto-cut" option is increasingly popular. This uses an apparently higher power setting but gives good control of tissue heating and cutting, because the system automatically adjusts power output according to initial

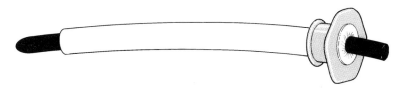

Fig 2.12 An overtube with biteguard over a rubber lavage tube.

tissue resistance and increasing resistance during coagulation and desiccation.

The type of current is generally less important than the amount of power produced, and other physical factors such as electrode pressure or snare-wire thickness and squeeze are more critical. High settings (high power) of coagulating current provide satisfactory cutting characteristics, whereas units with output not rated directly in watts can be assumed to have "cut" power output much greater than that of "coag" at the same setting. The difference in current type used is therefore often illusory. If in doubt, pure coagulating current alone is considered by most expert endoscopists to be safer and more predictable, giving "slow cook" effect and maximum hemostasis.

Lasers and argon plasma coagulation

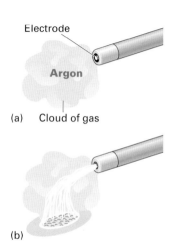

Electrode

Argon

(a)   Cloud of gas

(b)

Fig 2.13 Argon plasma coagulation (APC).

Lasers (particularly the neodymium-YAG and argon lasers) were introduced into endoscopy for treatment of bleeding ulcers, and for tumor ablation, because it seemed desirable to use a "no touch" technique. However, it has become clear that the same effects can be achieved with simpler devices, and that pressure (coaptation) may actually help hemostasis.

Argon plasma coagulation (*APC*) is easier to use and as effective as lasers for most endoscopic purposes. APC electrocoagulates, without tissue contact, by using the electrical conductivity of argon gas—a similar phenomenon to that seen in neon lights. The argon, passed down an electrode catheter (Fig 2.13a) and energized with an intelligent-circuitry electrosurgical unit and patient plate, ionizes to produce a local plasma arc—like a miniature lightning strike (Fig 2.13b). The heating effect is inherently superficial (2–3 mm at most, unless current is applied in the same place for many seconds), because tissue coagulation increases resistance and causes the plasma arc to jump elsewhere. However, APC action alone may be too superficial to debulk a larger lesion, requiring preliminary piecemeal snare-loop removal, with APC to electrocoagulate the base.

Equipment maintenance

Endoscopes are expensive and complex tools. They should be stored safely, hanging vertically in cupboards through which air can circulate. Care must be taken when carrying instruments, as the optics are easily damaged if left to dangle or are knocked against a hard surface. The head, tip, and umbilical cord should all be held (Fig 2.14).

The life of an endoscope is largely determined by the quality of maintenance. Complex accessories (e.g. electrosurgical equipment) must be checked and kept in safe condition. Close collaboration with hospital bioengineering departments and servicing engineers is essential. Repairs and maintenance must be properly documented.

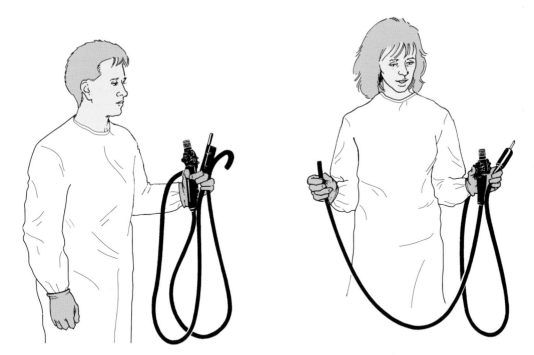

Fig 2.14 Carry endoscopes carefully to avoid knocks to the optics in the control head and tip.

Channel blockage

Blockage of the air/water (or suction) channel is one of the most common endoscope problems. Special "channel-flushing devices" are available, allowing separate syringe flushing of the air and water channels; they should be used routinely. When blockage occurs, the various systems and connections (instrument umbilical, water bottle cap or tube, etc.) must be checked, including the tightness and the presence of rubber O-rings where relevant. It is usually possible to clear the different channels by using the manufacturer's flushing device or a syringe with a suitable soft plastic introducer or micropipette tip. Water can be injected down any channel and, because water is not compressed, more force can be applied than with air. Remember that a small syringe (1–5 mL) generates more pressure than a large one, whereas a large one (50 mL) generates more suction. The air or suction connections at the umbilical, or the water tube within the water bottle, can be syringed until water emerges from the instrument tip. Care should be taken to cover or depress the relevant control valves while syringing. Another method for unclogging the suction channel is to remove the valve and apply suction directly at the port.

Infection control

There is a risk of transmitting infection in the endoscopy unit from patient to patient, patient to staff, and even from staff to patient.

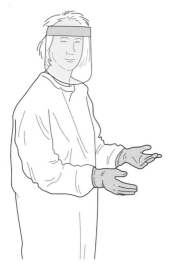

Fig 2.15 Gowns, gloves, and eye protection should be worn.

Universal precautions should always be adopted. This means assuming that all patients are infectious, even if there is no objective evidence. Infection control experts and equipment manufacturers should be welcomed as partners in minimizing infection risk; they should be invited to participate in developing unit policies and in monitoring their effectiveness through formal quality control processes. Infection control policies should be written down and understood by all staff.

Staff protection

Staff should be immunized against hepatitis; tuberculosis checks are mandatory in some units. Splashing with body fluids is a risk for staff in contact with patients and instruments. Gowns, gloves, and eye protection should be worn for these activities (Fig 2.15).

Other measures to reduce the risk of infection include:
* *frequent hand-washing*;
* *use of paper towels* when handling soiled accessories;
* disposal of *soiled items* directly into a sink or designated area (not on clean surfaces);
* *separate disposal of hazardous waste*, needles, and syringes;
* *covering skin breaks* with a waterproof dressing;
* *maintenance of good hygienic practice* throughout the unit.

Cleaning and disinfection

There are three levels of disinfection:
1 *Low-level disinfection* (essentially "wipe-down") is adequate for *non-critical accessories*, which come into contact with intact skin, e.g. cameras and endoscopic furniture.
2 *Sterilization* is required for *critical reusable accessories*, which enter body cavities and vasculature or penetrate mucous membranes, e.g. biopsy forceps, sclerotherapy needles, and sphincterotomes. "Single-use" disposable items are pre-sterilized.
3 *High-level disinfection* is required for *semi-critical accessories*, which come into contact with mucous membranes, e.g. endoscopes and esophageal dilators.

Endoscope reprocessing

Guidelines for cleaning and disinfecting endoscopes should be determined in each unit (and documented in the procedure manual) after consulting with manufacturers, infection control experts, and appropriate national advisory bodies. Endoscopists should be fully aware of their local practice, not least because they may be held legally responsible for any untoward event.

All advisory bodies require high-level disinfection of endoscopes and other equipment shortly after use.

How long a disinfected instrument remains fit for use after disinfection is an important issue, and still a matter for debate. Some authorities have recommended 4–7 days, but the reality depends on several factors. Endoscopes that contain retained moisture will rapidly become colonized by the rinsing water. Assiduous care must be taken in the drying process, and specially designed drying cabinets are available commercially. Local policy should be guided by national recommendations and can be validated by microbiological monitoring.

Formal cleaning and disinfection procedures should take place in a purpose-designed area. There should be clearly defined and separate clean and dirty areas, multiple worktops, and double sinks as well as a separate hand washbasin, endoscopic reprocessors (washing machines), and ultrasonic cleaners. An appropriately placed fume hood is also desirable.

Mechanical cleaning

The first and vitally important task in the disinfection process is to clean the endoscope and all of its channels, to remove all blood, secretions, and debris. Disinfectants cannot penetrate organic material.

Initial cleaning must be done immediately after the endoscope is removed from the patient.

1 *Wipe down* with a cloth soaked in enzymatic detergent.

2 *Suck water and enzymatic detergent* through the suction/biopsy channel, alternating with air, until the solution is visibly clean.

3 *Flush the air/water channel* with the manufacturer's flushing device or by depressing the air/water button while occluding the water bottle attachment at the light source and holding the tip of the scope under water. This should be continued until vigorous bubbling is seen.

4 *Attach the cap that protects the electrical connections*, and transfer the scope (in protective packaging to avoid contamination) to the designated cleaning area.

5 *Remove all valves and biopsy caps*.

6 *Test the scope for leaks*, particularly in the bending section, by pressurizing it with the leak-testing device and immersing the instrument in water. Angulate the bending section in its four directions while the instrument is under pressure to identify leaks in the distal rubber that are only obvious when it is stretched. Ensure all pressure is removed before disconnecting the leak tester.

7 *Totally immerse the instrument* in warm water and neutral detergent, and then wash the outside of the instrument thoroughly with a soft cloth.

8 *Brush the distal end* with a soft toothbrush, paying particular attention to the air/water outlet jet and any bridge/elevator.

9 *Clean the biopsy channel opening and suction port* using the port cleaning brush provided. Pass a clean channel-cleaning brush suitable for the instrument and channel size through the suction channel until it emerges clean (at least three times), cleaning the brush itself each time before reinsertion. Pass the cleaning brush from the suction channel opening in the other direction.

10 *Place the endoscope into a reprocessor* to complete cleaning and disinfection (or continue manually).

11 *Clean all instrument accessories* equally scrupulously, including the air/water and suction valves, water bottles, and cleaning brushes.

Manual cleaning

After brushing:

1 *Attach the manufacturer's cleaning adapters* to the suction, biopsy, and air/water channels. Ensure that the instrument remains immersed in the detergent fluid.

2 *Flush each channel with detergent* fluid, ensuring that it emerges from the distal end of each channel.

3 *Leave in detergent* for the time stated by the manufacturer of the detergent product used.

4 *Purge detergent from the channels.*

5 *Flush each channel with clean water* to rinse the detergent fluid.

6 *Rinse the exterior of the endoscope.*

7 *Check that all air is expelled from the channels.*

Manual disinfection

Soak the instrument and accessories (such as valves) in the chosen disinfectant for the recommended contact time.

Disinfectants

Glutaraldehyde has been the most popular agent. It can destroy viruses and bacteria within a few minutes, is non-corrosive (to endoscopes), and has a low surface tension, which aids penetration. The length of contact time needed for disinfection varies according to the type of gluteraldehyde used, and the temperature. Guidelines vary between countries, but 20 minutes is commonly recommended. More prolonged soaking may be required in cases of known or suspected mycobacterial disease.

Glutaraldehyde does carry the risk of sensitization, and can cause severe dermatitis, sinusitis, or asthma among exposed staff. The risk increases with increasing levels and duration of exposure. Medical-grade latex gloves, or nitrile rubber gloves, should be worn, with goggles and/or a face mask to protect against splashes. Closed system reprocessors and fume hoods/extraction fans are important. Reprocessors should be self-disinfecting. The concentration of disinfectant should be monitored.

Peracetic acid, chlorine dioxide, Sterox and other agents have also been used for endoscope disinfection.

A *sterile water supply* (special filters may be needed) helps to reduce the risk of nosocomial infections.

Rinsing, drying, and storing

Following disinfection, reprocessors rinse the instruments internally and externally to remove all traces of disinfectant, using the all-channel irrigator. The air, water, and suction channels (and flushing and forceps elevation channels if fitted) are perfused with 70% alcohol and dried with forced air before storage. This must be done for all endoscopes processed either manually or by automated reprocessor (some reprocessors have this function as part of the cycle). Bacteria multiply in a moist environment, and the importance of drying instruments after disinfection cannot be overemphasized. Instruments should be hung vertically in a well-ventilated cupboard.

Accessory devices

Diagnostic and therapeutic devices (such as biopsy forceps) are critical accessories, and must be sterile. Many are now disposable. Reusable accessories, such as water bottles, are autoclaved or gas sterilized.

Quality control of reprocessing

Records should be kept of the disinfection process for every endoscope, including who cleaned it, when, and how. Records that link the endoscope with which the patient was examined should also be kept. Routine bacteriological surveillance of automatic disinfectors and endoscopes is recommended by some experts, but is not yet endorsed by the main national societies, and is not widely practiced. This should allow early detection of serious contaminating organisms such as *Pseudomonas* and atypical mycobacteria. Routine surveillance also allows the early detection of otherwise unrecognizable internal channel damage, reprocessing protocol errors, as well as any water and environmental contamination problems. The specter of prion-related disease may be raised in patients with degenerative neurological symptoms. As prion proteins are not inactivated by heat or current disinfection regimes, disposable accessories should be used with a back-up endoscope reserved for such suspect patients. Lymphoid tissue is a particular risk, so many units now advise against routine ileal biopsies, particularly of Peyer's patches, for fear of potential prion contamination of the instrument channels.

Remember, although most of the cleaning, disinfection, and maintenance activities are normally and appropriately delegated to the staff, it is the endoscopist who is responsible for ensuring that their equipment is safe to use. Endoscopists should know how to complete the process themselves, especially in some emergency situations where the usual endoscopy nurses may not be available.

Safety and monitoring equipment

It is now standard practice to monitor patients through the procedural process and to provide supplemental oxygen in many cases. The necessary equipment must be readily available in the procedure rooms and pre-recovery areas, along with an emergency resuscitation cart.

Further reading

ASGE Quality Assurance In Endoscopy Committee, Petersen BT, Chennat J. Multisociety guideline on reprocessing flexible gastrointestinal endoscopes: 2011. *Gastrointest Endosc* 2011; **73**: 1075–84.

Beilenhoff U, Neumann CS, Rey JF *et al*. ESGE-ESGENA guideline: Cleaning and disinfection in gastrointestinal endoscopy. *Endoscopy* 2008; **40**: 939–7.

Guidelines for Decontamination of Equipment for Gastrointestinal Endoscopy Updated by: Dr Miles Allison—BSG Endoscopy Committee—February 2013 (available online at http://www.bsg.org.uk/clinical-guidelines/endoscopy/guidelines-for-decontamination-of-equipment-for-gastrointestinal-endoscopy.html).

Petersen BT, Chennat J, Cohen J *et al*. Multisociety guideline on reprocessing flexible GI endoscopes: 2011. *Infect Control Hosp Epidemiol* 2011; **32**: 527–37.

Rateb G, Sabbagh L, Rainoldi J *et al*. Reprocessing of endoscopes: results of an OMED-OMGE survey. *Can J Gastroenterol* 2005; WCOG abstracts. DR.1054. (available online at http://www.pulsus.com/WCOG/abs/DR .1054.htm).

Rutala WA, Weber DJ. Creutzfeldt–Jakob disease. Recommendations for disinfection and sterilization. *Clin Infect Dis* 2001; **32**: 1348–56.

US Society for Gastrointestinal Nurses and Assistants resource. (available online at http://infectioncontrol.sgna.org/SGNAInfectionPreventionRe sources/tabid/55/Default.aspx).

Willis C. Bacteria-free endoscopy rinse water—a realistic aim? *Epidemiol Infect* 2006; **134**: 279–84.

Now check your understanding—go to

www.wiley.com/go/cottonwilliams/practicalgastroenterology

CHAPTER 3

Patient Care, Risks, and Safety

Skilled endoscopists can now reach every part of the digestive tract and its appendages, such as the biliary tree and pancreas. It is possible to take specimens from all of these areas, and to treat many of their afflictions. Many patients have benefited greatly from endoscopy. Unfortunately, however, in some cases it may be an unhelpful procedure, and can even result in severe complications. There are also some hazards for the staff. The goal must be to maximize the benefits and minimize the risks. We need competent endoscopists, working for good indications on patients who are fully prepared and protected, with skilled assistants, and using optimum equipment. The basic principles are similar for all areas of gastrointestinal endoscopy, recognizing that there are specific circumstances where the risks are greater, including therapeutic and emergency procedures.

Patient assessment

Endoscopy is normally part of a comprehensive evaluation by a gastroenterologist or other digestive specialist. It is mostly used electively in the practice environment or hospital outpatient clinic, but sometimes may be needed in any part of a health-care facility (e.g. emergency room, intensive care unit, operating room). Sometimes endoscopists offer an "open access" service, where the initial clinical assessment and continuing care are performed by another physician. In all of these situations it is the responsibility of the endoscopist to ensure that the potential benefits exceed the potential risks, and personally to perform the necessary evaluations to make appropriate recommendations for the patient.

The following sections refer primarily to upper endoscopy. Issues specific to colonoscopy are covered in chapters 6 and 7.

Is the procedure indicated?

Upper endoscopy is now the primary tool for evaluating the esophagus, stomach, and duodenum. It may be used for many reasons. Broadly speaking, the goal may be to:

1 *make a diagnosis* in the presence of suggestive symptoms (e.g. dyspepsia, heartburn, dysphagia, anorexia, weight loss, hematemesis, anemia);

2 *clarify the status of a known disease* (e.g. varices, Barrett's esophagus);

Cotton and Williams' Practical Gastrointestinal Endoscopy: The Fundamentals, Seventh Edition.
Adam Haycock, Jonathan Cohen, Brian P Saunders, Peter B Cotton, and Christopher B Williams.
© 2014 John Wiley & Sons, Ltd. Published 2014 by John Wiley & Sons, Ltd.
Companion Website: www.wiley.com/go/cottonwilliams/practicalgastroenterology

3 *take specimens* (e.g. duodenal biopsy for malabsorption);
4 *screen for malignancy* and premalignancy in patients judged to be at increased risk of neoplasia (e.g. familial adenomatous polyposis);
5 *perform therapy* (e.g. hemostasis, dilatation, polypectomy, foreign body removal, tube placement, gastrostomy).

Several of the above indications may be combined: for example 1 and 5 (in acute bleeding), or 2 and 5 (e.g. retreatment of known varices).

Guidelines about the appropriate use of endoscopy are published by endoscopy organizations. The "strength" of the indication in each circumstance will depend upon likely benefit, the alternatives, and the perceived risks.

What are the risks? Unplanned events and complications

The vast majority of routine upper endoscopy procedures go according to plan, but there are exceptions. These may be generally categorized best as "unplanned events," which include technical failures (unable to reach the desired area) and clinical failures (no benefit from the treatment). Here we focus on adverse events. Some of these are relatively trivial, e.g. bleeding that stops without need for transfusion.

The term "complication" has unfortunate medicolegal connotations, so its use should be restricted to unplanned events of a certain defined level of severity. Over 15 years ago a group interested in the outcomes of endoscopic retrograde cholangiopancreatography (ERCP) proposed a definition that has been used widely ever since:

A complication is:
- an unplanned event;
- attributable to the procedure;
- that requires the patient to be admitted to hospital, or to stay longer than expected, or to undergo other interventions.

Levels of severity for complications

Complications can vary from relatively minor to life-threatening, so it is necessary to have some measure of severity. We use the degree of patient "disturbance" to stratify complications:
- *mild*—events requiring hospitalization of 1–3 days;
- *moderate*—hospital stay of 4–9 days;
- *severe*—stay of more than 10 days, or the need for surgery, or intensive care;
- *fatal*—death attributable to the procedure.

A multi-disciplinary working party of ASGE recently proposed a new lexicon for adverse events for all of the endoscopic procedures.

The new definition is: **An adverse event is an event that prevents completion of the planned procedure (not simply a technical failure or poor preparation or toleration), and/or results in a admission to hospital, prolongation of existing hospital stay, or another procedure (one requiring sedation/anesthesia), or subsequent consultation by another specialty.**

The working party also recommended allowing attribution to the events, (ie definite, probable, possible, unlikely).

Other publications from the working party included a detailed review of risk factors for events, and proposed new complexity scales for all endoscopic procedures.

Complication rates

Variable definitions and methods for data collection and a lack of community-based studies make it difficult to quote precise statistics about the risks of endoscopy, which obviously vary with the patient population and many other factors. However, large surveys suggest that the chance of suffering a severe complication (such as perforation or a major cardiopulmonary event) after ro utine upper endoscopy is less than 1 in 1000 cases. The risks are higher in the elderly and the acutely ill, and during therapeutic and emergency procedures. Inexperience, oversedation, and overconfidence are important factors.

Specific adverse events

• *Hypoxia* should be detected early by careful nursing surveillance, aided by pulse oximetry, and treated quickly.

• *Pulmonary aspiration* is probably more common than recognized. The risk is greater in patients with retained food residue (e.g. achalasia, pyloric stenosis), and in those with active bleeding.

• *Bleeding* may occur during and after endoscopy, from existing lesions (e.g. varices) or as a result of endoscopic manipulation (biopsy, polypectomy), or, occasionally, because of retching from a Mallory–Weiss tear. The risk of bleeding is greater in patients with coagulopathy, and in those taking anticoagulants and (possibly) antiplatelet agents.

• *Perforation* is the most feared complication of upper endoscopy. It is rare, most commonly occurs in the neck, and is more frequent in elderly patients, perhaps in the presence of a Zenker's diverticulum. The risk is minimized by gentle endoscope insertion under direct vision. Perforation beyond the cricopharyngeus is extremely unusual in patients who are not undergoing therapeutic techniques such as stricture dilatation, polypectomy, or mucosal resection. Perforation at colonoscopy is discussed in Chapter 7.

• *Cardiac dysrhythmias* are extremely rare. They require prompt recognition and expert treatment.

• *Intravenous (IV) site problems*. Many patients have discomfort at the site of their IV infusion. Local thrombosis is not unusual or dangerous, but evidence of spreading inflammation should be treated promptly and seriously.

• *Infection*. Patients with active infections can pose risks to the staff and to subsequent patients. Endoscopes (and accessories) are potential vehicles for the transmission of infection from patient to patient (e.g. *Helicobacter pylori*, salmonella, hepatitis, mycobacteria).

This risk should be eliminated by assiduous attention to detail in cleaning and disinfection. Endoscopy can provoke bacteremia, especially during therapeutic procedures such as dilatation. This may be dangerous in patients who are immunocompromised, and in some with diseased heart valves and prostheses. Endoscopy-induced endocarditis is extremely rare, but antibiotic prophylaxis is advised in certain circumstances (see below).

Assessing and reducing specific risks

Certain comorbidities and medications clearly increase the risk of endoscopic procedures. A *checklist* should be used to ensure that all of the issues have been addressed. Some of this information must be obtained when the procedure is scheduled, as action is required days ahead of the procedure (e.g. adjusting anticoagulants, stopping aspirin, etc.). Other aspects are dealt with when the patient arrives in the pre-procedure area.

• *Cardiac and pulmonary disease.* Patients with recent myocardial infarction, unstable angina, or hemodynamic instability are obviously at risk from any intervention. Expert advice should be sought from cardiologists. Endoscopy can be performed in patients with pacemakers and artificial implantable defibrillators, but the latter must be deactivated if diathermy is performed. Anesthetic supervision is essential if endoscopy is needed in such patients, and in others with respiratory insufficiency.

• *Coagulation disorders.* Patients with a known bleeding diathesis or coagulation disorder should have the situation normalized as far as possible before endoscopy (particularly if biopsy or polypectomy is likely). Anticoagulants can be stopped ahead of time, and (if clinically necessary) replaced by heparin for the period of the procedure, and early recovery. Certain antiplatelet drugs may need to be stopped also. There is little evidence that aspirin and nonsteroidal anti-inflammatory drugs (NSAIDs) increase the risk of adverse events. It is common practice, however, to ask about these drugs, and to recommend that they be discontinued for at least a week before endoscopic procedures.

• *Sedation issues.* Nervous patients and others who have had prior problems with sedation can pose challenges for safe endoscopy. Individuals who are at risk of airway obstruction (known sleep apnoea, obesity) or aspiration should undergo pre-endoscopy airway assessment. If in doubt, consider anesthesia support.

• *Endocarditis.* The risk of developing endocarditis after upper endoscopy procedures is extremely small, and there is no evidence that antibiotic prophylaxis is beneficial other than in percutaneous endoscopic gastrostomy (PEG) insertion and selectively for high-risk patients undergoing ERCP in which complete duct drainage is not successful. Current recommendations are made by national organizations (Table 3.1). The local policy should be documented in the endoscopy unit policy manual.

• *Pregnancy.* Endoscopy is generally safe to perform during pregnancy. Nonetheless, it should only be done when there is a strong indication and after consultation with an obstetrician. When possible, postponement to the second trimester is best.

Table 3.1 Antibiotic prophylaxis: policy at the Medical University of South Carolina. This is based on previous guidelines from the American Heart Association and the American Society for Gastrointestinal Endoscopy. Physician discretion is advised for other cardiac lesions (rheumatic valvular heart disease, acquired valvular dysfunction, mitral valve prolapse with insufficiency, hypertrophic cardiomyopathy, congenital malformations) and in patients having sclerotherapy or esophageal dilation. Special circumstances may justify other approaches. The final decision and responsibility rests with the endoscopist in each case

Endoscopies	Patient status	Regime	Alternative in case of allergy
All	Immunocompromised (neutrophils <1000, or transplant)	Cefotaxime 2 g IV	Clindamycin 900 mg IV and Aztreonam 1 g IV
Variceal treatment	Cirrhosis with ascites	Ofloxacin 200 mg IV over 1 h then 200 mg 12 hourly	–
PEG	All patients	Cefazolin 1 g IV	Vancomycin 1 g IV over 1 h

Table 3.2 ASA (American Society of Anesthesiologists) classification—anesthesia risk classes

Classification	Description	Example
Class I	Healthy patient	
Class II	Mild systemic disease—no functional limitations	Controlled hypertension, diabetes
Class III	Severe systemic disease—definite functional limitation	Brittle diabetic, frequent angina, myocardial infarction
Class IV	Severe systemic disease with acute, unstable symptoms	Recent myocardial infarction, congestive heart failure, acute renal failure, uncontrolled active asthma
Class V	Severe systemic disease with imminent risk of death	

The American Society of Anesthesiologists (ASA) score is used in many units to describe broad categories of fitness for procedures and sedation (Table 3.2). Many recommend anesthesia assistance for patients with ASA scores of 3 or greater.

Patient education and consent

Patients are entitled to be fully informed of the reasons why a procedure is recommended, the expected benefits, the potential risks, the limitations, and the alternatives. They also need to know exactly what will happen, and have the chance to ask questions.

Printed brochures can facilitate this education process and should be given (or sent) to patients well in advance of the procedure, so that they can be studied carefully and digested. Suitable brochures are available from national organizations, and on websites from expert centers (e.g. www.ddc.musc.edu). One example is shown in Fig 3.1. They can be adapted or developed for local conditions. Some centers use videotapes and web-based

Upper Endoscopy

Upper endoscopy is a test that lets your doctor see the lining of your upper digestive system. The upper digestive system includes the food tube (esophagus), the stomach and the first part of the small intestine (duodenum).

Upper endoscopy is the best way to find swelling (inflammation), ulcers or tumors of the upper digestive system.

Upper endoscopy can be used to treat some conditions present in the upper digestive system. Growths (polyps) and swallowed objects can be removed. Narrow areas can be stretched. Bleeding can be treated.

What is an Endoscope?

An endoscope is a long, narrow, flexible tube containing a tiny light and camera at one end.
This camera carries pictures of your upper digestive tract to a television screen. The doctor and nurse can see your esophagus, stomach, and small intestine better on this monitor. The pictures can also be recorded and printed.

How Do I Prepare?

Do not eat or drink for 6 hours before your test. Your stomach must be empty.

Tell your doctor if you...
• have any allergies, heart or lung problems.
• are or think you may be pregnant.
• have had endoscopy in the past and if you had problems with the medicines or dye used.
• take antibiotics before having dental work.

If you take medicine to thin your blood, (i.e. heparin or coumadin) or aspirin compounds tell your doctor. In general, you must stop taking these pills for several days, but in some cases you may continue to take them.

If you are a diabetic, please ask your doctor if you should take your insulin and/or pills before your test.

You may take blood pressure and heart medicine as usual the morning of your test.

If you take pills in the morning, drink only a small sip of water to help you swallow.

Do not take any antacids.

Bring with you all prescription and over-the-counter medicines you are taking.

Bring with you all medical records and X-ray films that relate to your current problem.

Make sure an adult can take you home. The medicines used during the procedure will not wear off for several hours. You will NOT be able to drive. If you travel by public transportation, such as by bus, van or taxi, you will still need an adult to ride home with you.

If you come alone, your test may have to be rescheduled.

Fig 3.1 MUSC patient education brochure (sedation is routinely used).

What Will Happen During My Upper Endoscopy?

1. When you come for the Upper Endoscopy, the doctor will talk to you about the test and answer any questions you have. You should know why you are having an Upper Endoscopy and understand the treatment options and possible risks.

2. You will put on a hospital gown. You will be asked to remove any eye glasses, contact lenses or dentures. An IV will be started and blood may be drawn for lab studies. You may receive antibiotics through the IV at this time.

3. You will be asked to sign a consent form which gives the doctor your permission to do the test.

4. You will be taken by stretcher to the procedure room. The nurse will help you get into the correct position, usually on your side, and make you comfortable. A medicine will be sprayed onto the back of your throat to make it numb. The medicine may taste unpleasant but it will stop any coughing during the test and the taste will go away quickly. A plastic guard will be placed in your mouth to protect your teeth during the test.

5. A blood pressure cuff will be put on your arm or leg. A small clip will be put on your finger. These will let the nurse check your blood pressure and heart rate frequently during the test.

6. If you require sedation, you will be given medicine through the IV. When you are relaxed and sleepy, the doctor will place a thin, flexible endoscope through the mouth guard and into your mouth. The endoscope has a small video camera on the end that lets the doctor see the inside of your esophagus.

7. The doctor will ask you to swallow. When you swallow, the endoscope will gently move down your esophagus, the same way food goes down when you are eating. You may feel like gagging, but you should not feel any pain. The endoscope will not interfere with your breathing.

8. The doctor will guide the endoscope through your stomach and into your small intestine. This will allow the doctor to see the lining of your upper digestive system and treat any problems that may be found.

9. When the test is done, the doctor will slowly take out the endoscope. Your Upper Endoscopy will last between 10 and 20 minutes.

What Will Happen Afterwards?

1. You will be taken to the recovery area. Your blood pressure and heart rate are watched while you rest. You will wake up in about 10 minutes to an hour if you have been sedated.

2. After removing your IV, the nurse will give you written instructions to follow when you go home. If you have any questions, please ask. The doctor will talk to you about your test before you leave.

3. Even if you feel awake, your judgment and reflexes will be slow. You may NOT be allowed to leave unless an adult takes you home. It is not safe for you to drive.

4. If treatments were done during your test, you may need to be observed overnight in hospital.

Fig 3.1 Continued.

5. If specimens were taken at your endoscopy, the results will be sent to you and the doctor who is providing your continuing care.

Over the Next 24 Hours....

You might need to take things quietly until the next day.

After the test, you may feel bloated and pass gas. This is normal and will go away in a few hours.

Your throat may be sore for a few days.

You may resume your regular diet and medications after the procedure.

Do not drive, operate machinery, sign legal documents or make important decisions.

Do not drink alcohol or take sleeping or nerve pills.

What are the Risks?

Upper Endoscopy is usually simple, but there are some risks, especially when treatments are done during the test.

A tender lump may form where the IV was placed. The lump may not go away for several weeks. You will need to call your doctor if redness, pain or swelling in this hand or arm lasts for more than two days.

The medicines may make you sick. You may have nausea, vomiting, hives, dry mouth, or a reddened face and neck.

Severe problems occur in less than one case in 500. These include chest and heart difficulties, bleeding, or tearing (perforation) of the digestive system. If any of these problems happen, you will have to stay in the hospital. Surgery may be needed.

Your doctor will discuss these risks with you.

Call the Doctor if You....

• have severe pain.
• vomit.
• pass or vomit blood.
• have chills and fever above 101 degrees.

If you have any problems, call your specialist. If it is after regular business hours, page the 'GI Doctor on Call' through the paging operator at ....
This information is provided as an educational service of the ......
The content is limited and is not a substitute for professional medical care.

Fig 3.1 Continued.

instructional materials. Patients must be given the opportunity to ask questions of the endoscopist before being invited to confirm their understanding and agreement to the procedure by signing the consent form. This document simply confirms that the patient truly understands and accepts what is being proposed, including the potential for harm.

The very simplicity and safety of upper endoscopy may tempt busy endoscopists to hurry the consent process, or to delegate it to others. That is not good medical practice, and carries medico-legal risk.

Physical preparation

Before upper endoscopy the patient should prepare by taking nothing by mouth for about 6 hours (usually overnight) and changing into a loose-fitting gown. A series of medical checks and actions to optimize the safety of the intervention are undertaken, including a general medical review, confirmation of current medication, assessment of vital signs and cardiopulmonary status, and attention to the many details concerning risks and risk reduction as detailed above. IV access should be established, preferably in the right arm or hand. Spectacles and dentures should be removed and stored safely. Consultation with a nurse is helpful with regards to adjustment of chronic medications the night before or on the morning of the procedure (e.g. insulin and antihypertensives).

Preparation for colonoscopy is covered in Chapter 6.

Monitoring

Although the endoscopist has overall responsibility, the endoscopy nurse is the practical guardian of the patient's safety and comfort. Nursing surveillance should be supplemented with monitoring devices, at least for pulse rate, blood pressure, and oxygen saturation. Supplemental oxygen is used routinely in many units, although some argue that this may mask hypoventilation, which is better detected by monitoring of carbon dioxide (capnography). Electrocardiographic monitoring is desirable for any patient with cardiac problems, and for prolonged complex procedures. Emergency drugs and equipment must be available nearby, and the endoscopist should be trained in resuscitation and life support.

Sedation and other medications are given by the endoscopist or by the nurse under supervision. The nurse should document this process carefully, along with the patient's vital signs, monitoring data and the patient's response.

Medications and sedation practice

Sedation practice varies widely around the world. In many countries, most routine (diagnostic) upper endoscopy is performed without any sedation, using only pharyngeal anesthesia. Although the avoidance of sedation has obvious advantages in terms of safety and fast recovery (e.g. patients can drive themselves home), many patients in the developed world expect and receive some degree of sedation/analgesia. Chapter 7 includes some discussion of sedation in general and specifically for colonoscopy.

Conscious sedation is intended to make unpleasant procedures tolerable for patients, while maintaining their ability to self-ventilate, maintain a clear airway, and respond to physical stimulation and verbal commands. Endoscopists giving conscious sedation must be fully familiar with the techniques and dosing. Many centers mandate specific training, and credentialing, for conscious sedation. The training is given by anesthesiologists. In contrast to conscious sedation, in *deep sedation* the patient cannot be easily aroused, and there may be partial or complete loss of protective reflexes, including the ability to maintain a patent airway. This level of sedation requires anesthesia supervision.

Sedation/analgesic agents (Table 3.3)
Anxiolytics
Short-acting benzodiazepines are commonly administered by slow IV injection/titration. Midazolam (Versed®), with its fast onset of action, short duration of action, and high amnestic properties, makes an ideal choice. It is given in an initial dose of 0.5–2.0 mg, with increments of 0.5–1 mg every 2–10 minutes, to a maximum of about 5 mg. Doses are determined by the patient's age, weight, medical and drug history, and by the response. Diazepam (Valium®, or in emulsion as Diazemuls®) can be used instead.

Table 3.3 Commonly used medication agents. For sedation purposes 25–50% increments of the initial dose can be administered every 2–10 minutes. Dosages should be adjusted according to patient age, body weight, medical history, and concomitant drug use

Sedating/ analgesic agents	Initial IV dose	Onset	Duration of effect
Midazolam	0.5–2 mg	1–5 min	1–2 h
Diazepam	1–5 mg	1–5 min	2–6 h
Meperidine	25–50 mg	2–5 min	2–4 h
Fentanyl	50–100 µg	1 min	20–60 min
Diphenhydramine	10–50 mg	1–10 min	2–6 h
Droperidol	1–5 mg	5–10 min	2–4 h
Reversal agents			
Flumazenil (for benzodiazepines)	0.1–0.2 mg	30–60 s	30–60 min
Naloxone (for opioids)	0.2–0.4 mg (IV and IM)	1–2 min	45 min

Narcotics

Narcotic analgesics are often given with benzodiazepines, but the combination increases the risk of respiratory depression. Pethidine (meperidine) is given in an initial dose of 25–50 mg, with increments of 25 mg up to a maximum of 100 mg. Fentanyl (Sublimaze®) is a more potent opioid analgesic with a rapid onset of action and clearance and reduced incidence of nausea compared with meperidine. It is useful in patients intolerant to meperidine but does have an increased risk of respiratory depression.

Antagonists

Meperidine can be reversed by naloxone, given both intramuscularly (IM) and intravenously (IV). Benzodiazepines are reversed by flumazenil, given by slow IV injection. Both antagonists have shorter half-lives than the drugs they antagonize.

Anesthesia

Although the vast majority of standard upper endoscopy procedures can be performed with endoscopist-directed sedation (or with no sedation), there are circumstances in which the presence of an anesthesiologist is helpful, and sometimes even full anesthesia is required. Examples include young children, heavy drinkers, patients who are difficult to sedate, and patients with high-risk cardiopulmonary status. Propofol (Diprivan®) is a useful short-acting anesthesia agent that seems ideal for endoscopy procedures. It has a weak amnestic effect and no analgesic effect and therefore is often used in conjunction with a short-acting opiate and benzodiazepine. In most centers and countries this can be given only by anesthesiologists.

Numerous other sedation/anesthesia practices have been tested and used, such as patient-controlled nitrous oxide and acupuncture.

Other medications

Pharyngeal anesthesia (given by spray) is used in many units to suppress the gag reflex during endoscopy. The patient should not be asked to say "ah" when applying the spray because this exposes the larynx to the anesthesia, which may suppress the cough reflex. Some endoscopists avoid local anesthesia when using sedation, believing that it may increase the risk of aspiration.

Excessive intestinal contraction can be suppressed with intravenous injections of **glucagon** (increments of 0.25 mg up to 2 mg) or **hyoscine butylbromide** (Buscopan®) 20–40 mg in countries where it is available.

Silicone-containing emulsions—either swallowed beforehand or injected down the channel—can be used to suppress foaming.

Pregnancy and lactation

Although this area has not been extensively studied, meperidine alone is preferred for procedural sedation during pregnancy.

Midazolam, although listed as category D by the US Food and Drug Administration, can be used in small doses in combination with meperidine as needed. If deep sedation is required it should performed by an anesthesiologist.

Concentrations of sedatives and analgesics vary in breast milk after procedural administration. In general, breast-feeding may be continued after fentanyl administration, which is preferred over meperidine during lactation. Infants should not be breast-fed for at least 4 hours following maternal administration of midazolam.

Recovery and discharge

After the endoscope is removed, the assisting nurse checks on the status of the patient and then transfers care to the recovery area staff. Monitoring is continued until the patient is fully awake, usually 20–30 minutes after standard sedation. A longer period of observation may be necessary after deep sedation or full general anesthesia.

The patient will appreciate a drink after sedation once any pharyngeal anesthesia has worn off. When established discharge criteria have been met, the patient gets dressed and is then taken to an interview area to discuss the findings and further care. Endoscopy is not complete until the patient has been counseled about the findings, their implications, and resulting plans. If sedation has been given, it is essential that this process takes place in the presence of an accompanying person, because of the potential for significant delayed amnesia. In addition, the patient should be instructed to have a responsible person to escort them home. They should not be allowed to drive, make important medicolegal decisions, or operate heavy machinery.

Discharge instructions should be given in writing, including details of:
• resumption of diet and activities;
• medications to be restarted, stopped, and commenced;
• further appointments;
• how biopsy results will be communicated;
• symptoms to report (and who to contact), including severe pain, distension, fever, vomiting, or passing blood.

Some units also print out and provide patient education materials relevant to the specific endoscopic findings. This service will become automatic with fully integrated electronic endoscopy reporting and management systems.

Managing an adverse event

Careful attention to all of these safeguards and cautions will help to ensure that most procedures go smoothly. Nevertheless, unplanned events do occur, even in the best of hands and environments, and it is natural for endoscopists and staff to feel bad when things "go wrong," especially when they are severe or life-threatening.

The most important action is to prepare for and manage these situations appropriately. The well-informed patient (and relatives) will have been told and should know that bad things can happen. This is an integral and important part of the communication and consent process, so it is appropriate and correct to address complications in that spirit. For example: "It looks like we have a perforation here. We discussed that as a remote possibility beforehand, and I'm sorry that it has occurred. This is what I think we should do."

Your distress is understandable and worthy, and you need to be sympathetic, but it is important also to be professional and matter of fact. Excessive apologies may give the impression that some avoidable mishap has occurred. Never attempt to cover up the facts. Document what has happened and communicate widely—with the patient, interested relatives, referring doctors, supervisors, and your risk management office.

Act quickly. Delay in managing complications is foolish and can be dangerous, both medically and legally. Get appropriate radiographs and lab studies, expert advice, and a surgical opinion (from a surgeon who understands the issues) for anything that might remotely require surgical intervention. Sometimes it may be wise to offer transfer of the patient to a colleague or to a larger center, but if this happens try to keep in touch and to show continuing interest and concern. Patients (and relatives) do not like to feel abandoned.

Further reading

Guidelines on indications, sedation, risks and risk reduction can be found at www.asge.org, www.bsg.org.uk, www.gastrohep.com, and many other sources.

ASGE working party reports on adverse events, risk factors and complexity.

Cotton PB, Eisen G, Aabakken L *et al.* A lexicon for endoscopic adverse events: report of an ASGE workshop. *GIE* 2010; **71**: 446–54.

Cotton PB, Eisen G, Romagnuolo J *et al.* Grading the complexity of endoscopioc procedures; results of an ASGE working party. *GIE* 2011; **73**: 868–74.

Romagnuolo J, Cotton PB, Eisen G *et al.* Identifying and reporting risk factors for adverse events in endoscopy. *GIE* 2011; **73**: 579–85 and 586–97.

Allison MC, Sandoe JAT, Tighe R, Simpson IA, Hall RJ, Elliott TSJ, Prepared on behalf of the Endoscopy Committee of the British Society of Gastroenterology. Antibiotic prophylaxis in gastrointestinal endoscopy 2009. (available online at http://www.bsg.org.uk/images/stories/docs/clinical/guidelines/endoscopy/prophylaxis_09.pdf).

American Society for Gastrointestinal Endoscopy. Quality safeguards for ambulatory gastrointestinal endoscopy. *Gastrointest Endosc* 1994; **40**: 799–800.

American Society for Gastrointestinal Endoscopy. Multisociety Sedation Curriculum for Gastrointestinal Endoscopy. *Gastrointest Endosc* 2012: **76**: e1–e25.

Axon ATR (ed.) *Infection in Endoscopy. Gastrointestinal Endoscopy Clinics of North America*, Vol. **3**(3) (series ed. Sivak MV). Philadelphia: WB Saunders, 1993.

Bell GD. Premedication, preparation and surveillance. *Endoscopy* 2002; **34**: 2–12.

Cooper GS. Indications and contraindications for upper gastrointestinal endoscopy. In: *Gastrointestinal Endoscopy Clinics of North America*, Vol. **4** (series ed. Sivak MV). Philadelphia: WB Saunders, 1994, pp. 439–54.

Cowen A. Infection and endoscopy: patient to patient transmission. In: Axon ATR (ed.) *Infection in Endoscopy. Gastrointestinal Endoscopy Clinics of North America*, Vol. **3**(3) (series ed. Sivak MV). Philadelphia: WB Saunders, 1993, pp. 483–96.

Dajani AS, Bison AL, Chung KL *et al*. Prevention of bacterial endocarditis: recommendations by the American Heart Association. *JAMA* 1990; **264**: 2919.

Plumeri PA. Informed consent for upper gastrointestinal endoscopy. In: *Gastrointestinal Endoscopy Clinics of North America*, Vol. **4** (series ed. Sivak MV). Philadelphia: WB Saunders, 1994; pp. 455–61.

Quine MA, Bell GD, McCloy RF, Charlton JE, Devlin HB, Hopkins A. Prospective audit of upper gastrointestinal endoscopy in two regions of England; safety, staffing, and sedation methods. *Gut* 1995; 462–7.

Royal College of Anaesthetists. *Implementing and Ensuring Safe Sedation Practice for Healthcare Procedures in Adults*. UK Academy of Medical Royal Colleges and their faculties. Report of an Intercollegiate Working Party chaired by the Royal College of Anaesthetists, 2002. (available online at www.rcoa.ac.uk).

Rutala WA, Weber DJ. Creutzfeldt–Jakob disease: recommendations for disinfection and sterilization. *Clin Infect Dis* 2001; **32**: 1348–56.

Shepherd H, Hewett D. *Guidance for Obtaining a Valid Consent for Elective Endoscopic Procedures*. A report of the Working Party of the British Society of Gastroenterology, 2008. (available online at http://www.bsg.org.uk/images/stories/docs/clinical/guidelines/endoscopy/consent08.pdf).

Teague R on behalf of the Endoscopy Section Committee of the British Society of Gastroenterology. Safety and sedation during endoscopic procedures. Update 2003. (available online at http://www.bsg.org.uk/images/stories/docs/clinical/guidelines/endoscopy/sedation.doc).

Now check your understanding—go to
www.wiley.com/go/cottonwilliams/practicalgastroenterology

CHAPTER 4

Upper Endoscopy: Diagnostic Techniques

Details of patient preparation are given in Chapter 3, along with some discussion of indications and risks. Both the endoscopist and the patient must be confident that the procedure is likely to be worthwhile and that it will be performed skillfully, with appropriate equipment and assistance.

Patient position

The patient lies on the examination trolley/stretcher on the **left** side with the intravenous access line preferably in the **right** arm. The height of the stretcher may be adjusted for comfort of the endoscopist. The patient's head is supported on a small, firm pillow, so as to remain in a comfortable neutral position (Fig 4.1).

Monitoring devices are attached and supplemental oxygen is given, usually via nasal prongs. Necessary sedation and/or pharyngeal anesthesia is applied. A biteguard is placed.

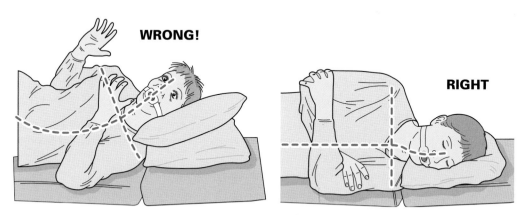

Fig 4.1 Preparing the patient correctly for upper gastrointestinal endoscopy.

Cotton and Williams' Practical Gastrointestinal Endoscopy: The Fundamentals, Seventh Edition.
Adam Haycock, Jonathan Cohen, Brian P Saunders, Peter B Cotton, and Christopher B Williams.
© 2014 John Wiley & Sons, Ltd. Published 2014 by John Wiley & Sons, Ltd.
Companion Website: www.wiley.com/go/cottonwilliams/practicalgastroenterology

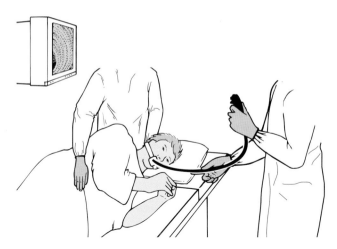

Fig 4.2 A confident and balanced stance with a straight instrument, gently handled.

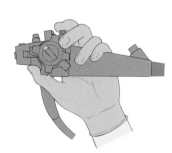

Fig 4.3 The thumb rests on the up/down angulation control with the forefinger on the air/water valve; the middle finger can also assist.

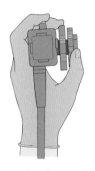

Fig 4.4 The thumb can reach across to the left/right control.

Endoscope handling

The endoscopist should stand comfortably facing the patient, holding the instrument so that it runs in a gentle curve to the patient's mouth (Fig 4.2).

The control head of the endoscope should be placed in the palm of the left hand and held between the fourth and fifth fingers and the base of the thumb, with the tip of the thumb resting on the up/down control (Fig 4.3). This grip leaves the first finger free to activate the air/water and suction buttons. The second finger assists the thumb as a helper or "ratchet" during major movements of the up/down control. Some people can also manage the left/right control with the left thumb (Fig 4.4). Twisting the control body applies torque to the straightened shaft and is an important part of steering.

The right hand is used to push and pull the instrument, to apply torque rotation and to control accessories such as biopsy forceps.

Passing the endoscope

Select a standard forward-viewing endoscope and check it. Perform a white-light balance (where necessary), lubricate the distal tip and double check the critical functions:
* tip angulation
* air and water
* suction
* image quality.

Check that the patient is stable and comfortable and that the assisting nurse is ready. Sedated, patients may slump into positions in which swallowing anything is a challenge. The patient should be facing directly in front, with the neck slightly flexed. Most endoscopists pass instruments under direct vision. Sometimes it may be necessary to insert the endoscope blindly, or with finger-guidance.

Direct vision insertion

Insertion under direct vision is the best and standard method.

1 *Hold the endoscope comfortably*—the head with the left hand, and the shaft with the right hand at the 30 cm mark.

2 *Rehearse up/down movements of the controls* to ensure that the tip will move in the correct longitudinal axis to follow the pharynx (Fig 4.5). Adjust the lateral angulation control or twist the shaft appropriately so that the scope will travel down the midline.

3 *Pass the tip of the endoscope through the biteguard and over the tongue*, initially looking at the patient, not at the monitor.

4 Gently angle the tip "up" (with your left thumb on the angulation control) as it passes over the tongue.

5 *Now look at the monitor*. Due to the looping of the endoscope, the view is inverted. Look for a rough, pale surface of the tongue horizontally in the upper (anterior) part of the view and keep the interface between it and the red surface of the palate in the centre of view by angling up appropriately, while advancing inward over the curve of the tongue.

6 *Stay in the midline* by watching for the linear "median raphe" of the tongue or the convexity of its midpart (Fig 4.6a), correcting if necessary by twisting the shaft. The uvula is often seen transiently, projected *upward* in the lower part of the view (Fig 4.6b).

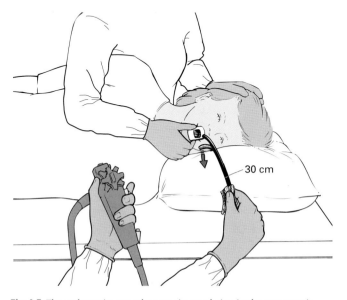

30 cm

Fig 4.5 The endoscopist pre-rehearses tip angulation in the correct axis before insertion.

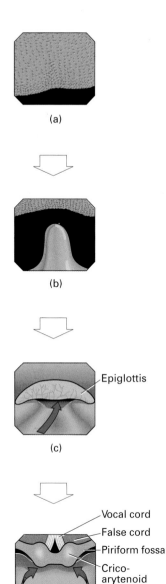

(a)

(b)

Epiglottis

(c)

Vocal cord

False cord

Piriform fossa

Crico-
arytenoid
cartilage

(d)

Fig 4.6 (a) Follow the centre of the tongue . . . (b) . . . past the uvula . . . (c) . . . and the epiglottis . . . (d) . . . to pass below the cricoarytenoid on either side.

7 *Advance gently*. The epiglottis and then the cricoarytenoid cartilage with the "false" vocal cords above it (and the vocal cords 2–3 cm beyond) are visible in the upper part of the view (Fig 4.6c).

8 The first, or pharyngeal, part of the esophagus is in tonic contraction and so is seen only transiently during swallowing. To reach it, angle downward (posteriorly) so that the tip passes inferior to the curve of the cricoarytenoid cartilage, preferably passing to one or other side of the midline as the midline bulge of the cartilage against the cervical spine makes central passage difficult (Fig 4.6d), and push inward.

9 *There is often a "red-out"* as the tip impacts into the cricopharyngeal sphincter; insufflate air, maintain **gentle** inward pressure, ask the patient to swallow, and the instrument should slip into the esophagus within a few seconds. If necessary, ask the patient to swallow again, pushing gently as the sphincter opens.

10 *Keep watching carefully* to ensure smooth mucosal "slide-by" as the instrument passes semi-blind into the upper esophagus, for this is where a diverticulum may occur.

11 Throughout this process:
  • *be gentle*, feel the tube slide in
  • coordinate gentle onward pressure with the patient's attempts to swallow
  • *encourage the patient*, e.g. "swallow, swallow again, well done . . . now take deep breaths." This is best done by the endoscopist alone. Too many voices may confuse the patient and may suggest a degree of panic.

12 If the view is lost, or a bulging tongue deflects the scope, or the teeth are seen, withdraw and start again.

13 *Be gentle*; force is dangerous and unnecessary (Video 4.1).

Blind insertion

This technique (originating from the time when most gastroscopes were side-viewing and were still used for endoscopic retrograde cholangiopancreatography (ERCP) insertions) is a slight variation of the better direct vision method but is done mainly by feel and by watching the patient, rather than looking at the endoscopic view on the monitor. The assistant maintains the patient's neck slightly flexed. The endoscopist passes the instrument tip through the biteguard and over the tongue to the back of the mouth; using the left thumb on the control knob, the tip is then actively deflected "upward" so that it curls in the midline over the back of the tongue and into the midline of the pharynx. The tip is advanced slightly and angled down a little, and the thumb is then removed from the tip control. Slight forward pressure is maintained, and the patient is asked to swallow as the 20 cm mark approaches the biteguard. There is an obvious feeling of "give" as the tip passes the cricopharyngeal sphincter and then slides easily into the esophagus.

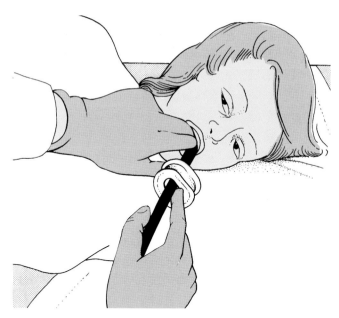

Fig 4.7 Sometimes "blind" insertion is helped by guiding the instrument between two fingers.

Insertion with tubes in place

Endotracheal tubes present no problem for the endoscopist inserting under direct vision, the scope being angled down posterior to the tube and gently pushed through the sphincter. Deflating the cuff of the tube may be necessary occasionally to allow easier passage, especially with larger instruments. An existing nasogastric tube may be a useful guide to the lumen. Withdrawing the endoscope may displace a nasogastric or nasoenteric tube. This risk can be minimized by stiffening the tube with a guidewire.

Finger-assisted insertion

This method is inelegant, and is needed only rarely when standard methods fail. The control head of the instrument is held by an assistant (avoiding contact with the angulation controls). The biteguard is fitted over the shaft before insertion. The endoscopist puts the second and third fingers of the left hand over the back of the tongue. With the right hand, the tip of the instrument is passed over the tongue, and the inserted fingers of the left hand are used to guide it into the midline of the pharynx (Fig 4.7). The fingers are withdrawn, the biteguard is slid into place, and the patient is asked to swallow. If swallowing is not effective, the tip of the instrument has probably fallen into the left pyriform fossa.

Routine diagnostic survey

Whatever the precise indication, it is usually appropriate to examine the entire esophagus, stomach, and proximal duodenum, wherever possible. A complete survey may sometimes be prevented by stricturing from disease or previous surgery, or can be curtailed for other reasons.

It is important to develop a systematic routine to reduce the possibility of missing any area.

• *Always advance the instrument under direct vision*, using air insufflation and suction as required, and slowing as necessary during active peristalsis.

• *Mucosal views are often optimal during instrument withdrawal*, when the organs are fully distended with air, but inspection during insertion is also important, as minor trauma by the instrument tip (or excessive suction) may produce small mucosal lesions with consequent diagnostic confusion.

• *Lesions noted during insertion are best examined in detail* (and sampled for histology or cytology) following a complete routine survey of other areas.

• *As well as being systematic in survey, be precise in movements and decisive in making a "mental map"* of what is being seen. A careful and complete examination can be achieved in less than 5–10 minutes by avoiding unnecessary movements and repeated examinations of the same area.

Golden rules for endoscopic safety:

• *do not push if you cannot see*
• *if in doubt, inflate and pull back*.

Esophagus

The esophagus (Fig 4.8) extends:

• from the cricopharyngeal sphinctert
• behind the left main bronchus, the left atrium and aorta
• to the esophagogastric mucosal junction, which is usually easy to see at 38–40 cm from the incisor teeth (in adults) as the point

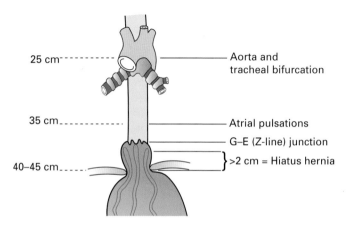

25 cm .... — Aorta and tracheal bifurcation

35 cm .... — Atrial pulsations
— G–E (Z-line) junction
40–45 cm ..... } >2 cm = Hiatus hernia

Fig 4.8 Esophageal landmarks—with a small hiatal hernia.

where pale pink squamous esophageal mucosa abuts darker red columnar gastric mucosa. This squamocolumnar junction is often irregular and therefore can also be called the "Z-line." The esophagogastric junction should be situated at the top of the gastric folds in a semi-inflated esophagus. Pink mucosa extending cephalad from the top of the gastric folds suggests Barrett's esophagus, biopsies being required to establish the diagnosis and exclude dysplasia.

The diaphragmatic hiatus normally clasps the esophagus at or just below the esophagogastric junction. The position of the hiatus can be highlighted by asking the patient to sniff or to take deep breaths, and is recorded as the distance from the incisors. In any patient, the precise relationship of the Z-line to the diaphragmatic hiatus varies somewhat during an endoscopy (depending on the patient position, respiration, and gastric distension). In normal patients, the gastric mucosa is often seen up to 1 cm above the diaphragm. A *hiatus hernia* is diagnosed if the Z-line remains more than 2 cm above the hiatus. From the clinical point of view, however, the presence or degree of herniation may be less important than any resulting esophageal lesions (e.g. esophagitis or the columnar transformation of Barrett's).

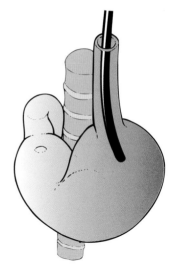

Fig 4.9 The distal esophagus angles the scope into the posterior wall of the lesser curve.

Stomach

In the absence of stenosis, the endoscope can be advanced easily through the cardia and into the stomach under direct vision. The distal esophagus usually angles to the patient's left as it passes through the diaphragm, so it may be necessary to turn the instrument tip slightly to remain in the correct axis (Fig 4.9). Unless the cardia is unduly lax, the mucosal view is lost momentarily as the tip passes through, passage being felt by the advancing hand as a slight "give." If the tip is further advanced in the same plane, it will abut on the posterior wall of the lesser curvature of the stomach, so that pushing in blindly risks retroflexing toward the cardia. Thus:

1 *rotate to the "left" (counterclockwise) to avoid the lesser curve*, and add air as the endoscope tip passes through the cardia

2 *if there is no clear luminal view, withdraw slightly* to disimpact the tip from the wall of the fundus or from the pool of gastric juice on the greater curve

3 *the endoscopic view is predictable* with the patient in the left lateral position and the instrument held correctly (buttons up) (Figs 4.10 and 4.11); the smooth lesser curvature is on the endoscopist's right with the angulus distally, the longitudinal folds of the greater curve are to the left and its posterior aspect is below

4 *aspirate any pool of gastric juice* to avoid reflux or aspiration during the procedure

5 *insufflate the stomach* enough to obtain a reasonable view during insertion

6 *inject a suspension of silicone* (simethicone) down the biopsy channel if there is excessive foaming.

The four walls of the stomach are examined sequentially by a combination of tip deflection, instrument rotation and advance/withdrawal. The field of view during the advance of a four-way

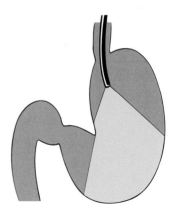

Fig 4.10 With the gastroscope high on the lesser curve . . .

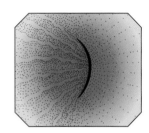

Fig 4.11 . . . the view is of the angulus in the distance, with the greater curve longitudinal folds. A fluid pool is often on the left.

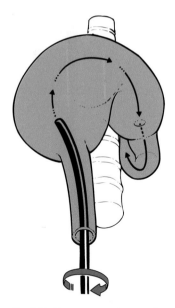

Fig 4.12 The route to pylorus and duodenum is a clockwise spiral around the vertebral column.

angling endoscope can be represented as a cylinder angulated over the vertebral bodies. The distended stomach takes up an exaggerated J-shape with the axis of the advancing instrument corkscrewing clockwise up and over the spine, following the greater curvature (Fig 4.12).

Thus, to advance through the stomach and into the antrum:
1 *angle the tip up increasingly*
2 *rotate the shaft clockwise*.

This clockwise corkscrew rotation through approximately 90° during insertion brings the angulus and antrum into end-on view (Fig 4.13). It may be necessary now to deflect the tip a little downward to bring it into the axis of the antrum (Fig 4.14), so that it runs smoothly along its greater curve. The motor activity of the antrum, pyloric canal, and pyloric ring should be carefully observed. Asymmetry during a peristaltic wave is a useful indicator of present or previous disease.

Through the pylorus into the duodenum

The pyloric ring is approached directly for passage into the duodenum. During the maneuver it is convenient to use only the left-hand for tip angulation and torque to maintain the instrument tip in the correct axis.

1 *Advance with the pyloric ring in the center of the view*. Passage is both felt and seen. Entry into the duodenal bulb is recognized by its granular and pale surface (Figs 4.15, 4.16 and 4.17).

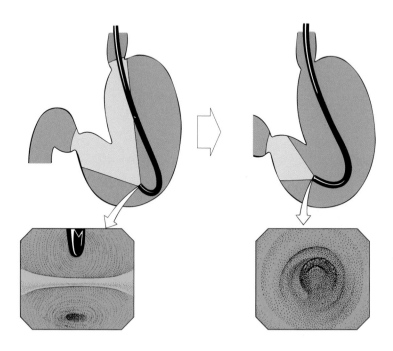

Fig 4.13 The angulus and antrum come into view . . .

Fig 4.14 . . . then angle down to see the pylorus in the axis of the antrum.

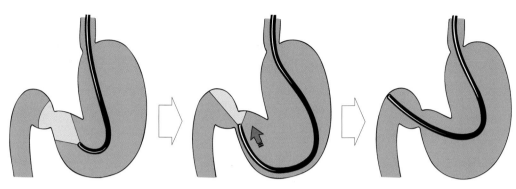

Fig 4.15 The scope passes from the antrum . . .

Fig 4.16 . . . to the pylorus and duodenal cap . . .

Fig 4.17 . . . and tends to impact in the duodenum.

2 Patience may be needed to pass the pylorus, especially if there is spasm or deformity; ***downward*** angulation of the tip or deflation may help its passage. As the instrument tip passes the resistance of the pylorus, the loop that has inevitably developed in the stomach straightens out and accelerates the tip to the distal bulb (Fig 4.17).
3 So, to obtain optimal views of the duodenal bulb, ***withdraw a few centimeters to disimpact the tip and insufflate some air*** (Fig 4.18).
4 ***Examine the bulb by circumferential manipulation of the tip*** during advance and withdrawal. The area immediately beyond the pyloric ring, especially the inferior part of the bulb, may be missed by the inexperienced, who fail to withdraw sufficiently for fear of falling back into the stomach.
5 ***Give an antispasmodic*** (Buscopan® or glucagon) intravenously if visualization is impaired by duodenal motility.
6 ***Avoid excessive air insufflation***, which will leave the patient uncomfortably distended.

Passage into the descending duodenum

The superior duodenal angle is the key landmark (Fig 4.18) connecting the bulb and the descending duodenum. To pass into the descending duodenum, *gently*:
1 *advance so that the tip lies at the angle*
2 *rotate the shaft about 90° to the right*
3 *angle to the right*
4 *angle up*.

This maneuver creates a corkscrew motion around the angle (Fig 4.19), and provides a tunnel view of the descending duodenum. Now, to advance further ***do not just push, as this will simply form a big loop in the stomach (Fig 4.20).*** Rather, it is necessary to ***pull back***. Straightening the loop in the stomach propels the tip onward, and the straightening shaft also corkscrews more efficiently round the superior duodenal angle (Figs 4.21 and 4.22). Using the correct "pull and twist" method, the tip slides in to reach the region of the major papilla with only about 60 cm of instrument inserted. A forward-viewing instrument gives tangential and often restricted views of the convex medial wall of the descending

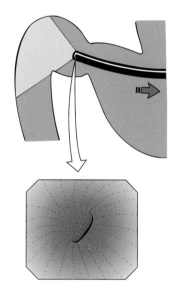

Fig 4.18 Withdraw the scope to disimpact the tip and see the superior duodenal angle—an important landmark.

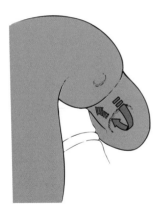

Fig 4.19 Corkscrew the tip clockwise around the superior duodenal angle, using twist, right, and up angulation simultaneously.

duodenum and the papilla. Much better views of this area are obtained with side-viewing instruments.

Retroflexion in the stomach (J maneuver)

The fundus of the stomach is often best seen in retroversion, i.e. from below. To achieve this view safely:

1 *place the tip of the endoscope in the mid stomach*, at or just beyond the angulus

2 *insufflate air*

3 *angle up acutely 180°* (using both angulation controls); this maneuver should demonstrate the angulus, the entire lesser curve and the fundus as the instrument is withdrawn (Fig 4.23)

4 *pull back slowly and rotate the shaft* to obtain complete views of the fundus and cardia (Fig 4.24); rotating the small dial to the maximal extent in both directions can aid in viewing the cardia

5 *do not pull back too far*, as this risks impacting the retroverted tip in the distal esophagus

6 *after retroversion, remember to return the angulation controls to the neutral position*.

Retroversion in the stomach is probably best performed after examining the duodenum so as to avoid overinflation on the way in. Some patients (particularly those with a lax cardia) find it difficult to hold enough air to permit an adequate view. If retroversion proves difficult, it may be made easier by rotating the patient slightly onto his or her back to give the stomach more room to expand.

During all of these maneuvers, it is helpful to keep the shaft of the instrument relatively straight from the patient's teeth to your hands. This reduces the strain on the endoscope, helps orientation, and ensures that your rotating movements are precisely transmitted to the tip.

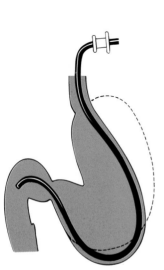

Fig 4.20 Because of the loop in the greater curve . . .

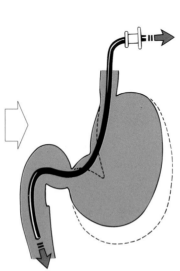

Fig 4.21 . . . withdrawal helps to advance the scope into the second part of the duodenum.

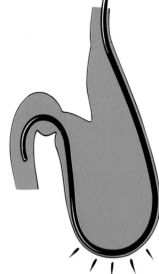

Fig 4.22 Trying to reach the third part by force simply forms a loop in the stomach.

Removing the instrument

The mucosa should be surveyed carefully once again during withdrawal. Under the different motility conditions and organ shapes produced by distension and instrument position, areas previously seen only tangentially on insertion may be brought into direct view on the way out. The proximal lesser curve, a potential "blind spot," merits particular attention as the scope withdraws along it. Remember to aspirate air (and fluid) from the stomach completely on withdrawal, and to release the brakes from the angulation controls (if they have been applied) (Video 4.2).

Finally, take a few seconds to reassure the patient, "Well done, it's all over, we will talk in a few minutes. . . ."

Now begin the cleaning process! It is important not to let blood and secretions dry on the instrument or in the channels. So, immediately:

1 *wipe the endoscope with a wet cloth*
2 *place the tip in water and depress both control valves* (to flush out any mucus or blood form the air/water channel and wash through the instrumentation channel)
3 *hand the instrument to the nurse/assistant* to start the cleaning and disinfection process.

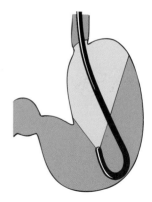

Fig 4.23 Angulation of 180° retroflexes the tip to see the lesser curve . . .

Problems during endoscopy

Patient distress

Endoscopy should be terminated quickly if the patient shows distress for which the cause is not immediately obvious and remediable. If reassurance does not calm the patient, remove the instrument and consider giving additional sedation or analgesia. Inadvertent bronchoscopy can occur if insertion is done by the "blind" method, and it is obvious from the unusual view and impressive coughing. Discomfort may arise from inappropriate pressure during intubation or from distension due to excessive air insufflation. Remember to keep inflation to a minimum and to aspirate all the air at the end of the procedure. Severe pain during endoscopy is very rare and indicates a complication such as perforation or a cardiac incident. It is extremely dangerous to ignore warning signs. Tachycardia and bradycardia may both indicate distress.

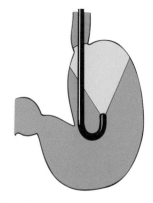

Fig 4.24 . . . and swinging the retroflexed tip around gives a view of the fundus and cardia.

Getting lost

The endoscopist may become disorientated and the instrument looped in patients with congenital malrotations or major pathology (e.g. achalasia, large diverticula, hernias) or after complex surgery. Careful study of any available radiographs may help. The commonest reason for disorientation in patients with normal anatomy is inadequate air insufflation due to a defect in the instrument or air pump (which should have been detected before starting the examination). Inexperienced endoscopists often get lost in the fundus, especially when the stomach is angled acutely over the vertebral column. Having passed the cardia, the instrument tip should be deflected to the endoscopist's *left* and slightly downward (Fig 4.25).

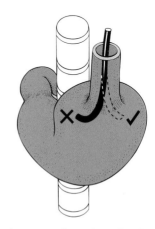

Fig 4.25 Angling right (rather than left) on entering the fundus can cause retroflexion and can result in getting lost.

A wrong turn to the right will bring the tip back up into the fundus. When in doubt, withdraw, insufflate, and turn sharply left to find the true lumen. A curious endoscopic view may indicate perforation (which is not always immediately painful). If in any doubt, abandon the examination and obtain radiological studies.

Inadequate mucosal view

Lack of a clear view means that the lens is lying against the mucosa or is obscured by fluid or food debris. Withdraw slightly and insufflate air; double check that the air pump is working and that all connections are firm with O-rings present. Try washing the lens with the normal finger-controlled water jet. This may not be effective if the instrument lens is covered by debris (or by mucosa that has been sucked onto the orifice of the biopsy channel). Pressure can be released by brief removal of the rubber valve of the biopsy port, but it may be necessary to flush the channel with water or air using a syringe. Small quantities of food or mucus obscuring an area of interest can be washed away with a jet of water. Foaming can be suppressed by adding a diluted emulsion of silicone (simethicone).

As most patients comply with instructions to fast before procedures, the presence of excessive food residue is an important sign of outlet obstruction. Standard endoscope channels are too small for aspiration of food; prolonged attempts simply result in blocked channels. The instrument can usually be guided along the lesser curvature over the top of the food to allow a search for a distal obstructing lesion. The greater curvature can also be examined if necessary by rotating the patient into the right lateral position. However, any examination in the presence of excess fluid or food carries a significant risk of regurgitation and pulmonary aspiration. The endoscopist should persist only if the immediate benefits are thought to justify the risk. It is usually wiser to stop and to repeat the examination only after proper gastric lavage.

Recognition of lesions

This book is concerned mainly with techniques, rather than with lesions. Several excellent atlases are available. However, certain points are worth emphasizing here.

Esophagus
Esophagitis
Esophagitis normally follows acid reflux and is most apparent distally, close to the mucosal junction. If the distal esophagus is normal with areas of inflammation in the mid or proximal esophagus, the cause is probably not due to reflux (drug or viral causes). There is no clear macroscopic dividing line from normality, the earliest visible reflux changes consisting of mucosal congestion and edema that obscure the normal fine vascular pattern, progressing to short breaks in the surface of the longitudinal esophageal folds (Fig 4.26), leading in more severe grades (Los Angeles classification) to longer linear breaks, then damage that is confluent or extends circumfer-

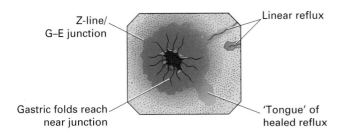

Fig 4.26 Minor reflux changes above hiatus hernia—no need for biopsies.

entially. The process culminates in symmetrical stricturing, above which the mucosa (now protected from reflux) may appear almost normal.

Barrett's esophagus

Barrett's esophagus is a potentially precancerous consequence of longstanding reflux damage. Red gastric-type mucosa is seen endoscopically to extend proximally from the top of the gastric folds in a semi-inflated esophagus. The pattern of this columnar extension may be in "tongues" or "circumferential" (or both), sometimes with columnar "islands" proximal to that. The maximum extent (in centimeters) of tongues or circumferential change should each be recorded. Quadrantic biopsies are taken every 2 cm circumferentially and from tongues or islands, looking for "specialized intestinal metaplasia" (Barrett's epithelium) and for any dysplasia within it (Fig 4.27). As long as no dysplasia is present, surveillance endoscopies can be performed every 2–5 years.

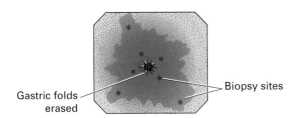

Fig 4.27 Barrett's esophagus—take biopsies.

Esophageal carcinoma

Esophageal carcinoma usually causes asymmetrical stenosis, with areas of exuberant abnormal mucosa and sometimes an irregular ulcer with raised edges. Carcinoma of the gastric fundus may also infiltrate upward submucosally to involve the esophagus. The correct diagnosis is then easily made if the endoscope can be passed through the stricture to allow retroverted views of the cardia.

Diverticula

Diverticula in the mid- or distal esophagus are easily recognized, but the instrument may enter a pulsion diverticulum (Zenker's) or pouch in the upper esophagus without the true lumen being seen at all. Lack of view and resistance to inward movement are (as always) an indication to pull back and reassess. Diverticula found in the mid-esophagus are caused by inflammatory swelling and subsequent contraction of subcarinal lymph nodes. These are termed "traction diverticula." Webs or rings, such as the Schatzki ring, at or just proximal to the esophagogastric junction may not be obvious to the endoscopist because of a combination of "flat" bright endoscope illumination and distortion from the wide-angled lens view.

Varices

Varices lie in the long axis of the esophagus as tortuous bluish mounds covered with relatively normal mucosa. They resemble varicose veins elsewhere in the body.

Mallory–Weiss tears

Mallory–Weiss tears are 5–20 mm longitudinal mucosal splits lying either side of or across the esophagogastric mucosal junction. These are thought to be caused by retching, but a history of this can be elicited in only 50% of cases. In the acute phase the tear is covered with exudate or clot and may sometimes be seen best in a retro-verted view.

Motility disturbances

Motility disturbances of the esophagus should be diagnosed by radiology and manometry, but their consequences—such as dilation, pseudodiverticula, food retention, and esophagitis—are well seen at endoscopy, which is always needed to rule out obstructing pathology.

Achalasia typically appears as a dilated, fluid-filled esophagus with ineffective or absent peristalsis. The endoscope passes easily through the lower esophageal sphincter and into the cardia, in contrast to the fixed narrowing of pathological strictures due to reflux esophagitis or malignancy.

Stomach

The appearance of the normal gastric mucosa varies considerably. Reddening (hyperaemia) may be generalized (e.g. with bile reflux into the operated stomach) or localized. Sometimes it occurs in long streaks along the ridges of mucosal folds. Localized (traumatic) reddening with or without petechiae or edematous changes is often seen on the posterior upper lesser curve in patients who habitually retch. Macroscopic congestion does not correlate well with underlying histological gastritis, and care should be taken when considering clinical relevance. Biopsy samples should be taken when any abnormality is suspected, and tests for *Helicobacter pylori* performed in patients with dyspepsia with or without macroscopic lesions.

Gastric folds

Gastric folds vary in size, but the endoscopic assessment also depends upon the degree of gastric distension. Very prominent fleshy folds are seen in Ménétrier's disease and are best diagnosed by a snare loop biopsy. Patients with duodenal ulceration often have large gastric folds with spotty areas of congestion within the areae gastricae and excess quantities of clear resting juice. With gastric atrophy, there are no mucosal folds (when the stomach is distended) and blood vessels are easily seen through the pale atrophic mucosa. Atrophy is often associated with intestinal metaplasia, which appears as small, gray-white plaques.

Erosions and ulcers

Erosions and ulcers are the most common localized gastric lesions. A lesion is usually called an erosion if it is small (<5 mm diameter) and shallow, with no sign of scarring. Acute ulcers and erosions are often seen in the antrum and may be capped with, and partially obscured by, clots. Edematous erosions appear as small, smooth, umbilicated raised areas, often in chains along the folds of the gastric body. "Gastritis" is a term best reserved for histological use.

The classic chronic benign gastric ulcer is usually single and is most frequently seen on the lesser curvature at or above the angulus. It is typically symmetrical with smooth margins and a clean base (unless eroding adjacent structures). Multiple and punched out ulcers (sometimes oddly shaped and very large) occur in some patients taking nonsteroidal anti-inflammatory drugs (NSAIDs).

Malignancy

Malignancy may be suspected if an ulcer has raised irregular margins (or different heights around the circumference), a lumpy hemorrhagic base or a mucosal abnormality surrounding the ulcer. Mucosal folds around a benign ulcer usually radiate toward it and reach the margin. At times it may be difficult to separate benign from malignant ulcers on macroscopic appearance alone; if there is doubt, tissue specimens should be taken from the ulcer edge. Unfortunately, gastric cancer is usually diagnosed at an advanced stage in Western countries, when it is all too obvious at endoscopy. Diffusely infiltrating carcinoma (*linitis plastica*) may be missed unless motility is carefully studied. Standard mucosal biopsies may be normal and a high degree of suspicion is required. Endoscopic ultrasonography (EUS) is the best method of differentiating the cause of enlarged gastric folds.

Early gastric cancer may mimic a small benign ulcer, chronic erosion, or a flat polyp. Polypoid lesions under 1 cm in diameter are usually benign in origin. However, as all malignant lesions start small and are curable if detected at an early stage, odd mucosal lumps and bumps should never be ignored; a tissue diagnosis must be made. Submucosal tumors are characterized by normal overlying mucosa and bridging folds; leiomyomas and plaques of aberrant pancreatic tissue (characteristically found in the floor of the antrum) usually have a central dimple or crater.

Duodenum
Duodenal ulcers

Duodenal ulcers, either current or previous, often cause persistent deformity of the duodenal bulb and/or pyloric ring. The ulcers occur most commonly on the anterior and posterior walls of the bulb and are frequently multiple. When active they are surrounded by edema and acute congestion. Scarring often results in a characteristic shelf-like deformity, which partially divides the bulb and may produce a pseudodiverticulum. A small linear ulcer or scar can be seen running along the apex of this fold. The mucosa of the bulb often reveals small mucosal changes of dubious clinical significance. Areas of mucosal congestion with spotty white exudate ("pepper and salt" ulceration) merge into even less definite macroscopic appearances labeled as "duodenitis." Small mucosal lumps in the proximal duodenum usually reflect underlying Brunner's gland hyperplasia or gastric metaplasia (ectopic islands of gastric mucosa). Duodenal tumors occur mainly in the region of the papilla of Vater.

Ulceration and duodenitis in the second part of the duodenum suggests Zollinger–Ellison syndrome or underlying pancreatic disease. Crohn's disease may be suspected by the presence of small aphthous ulcers in the second part; typical granulomas may be seen on histology.

Celiac disease

Celiac disease is now known to be significantly more common than previously thought. The characteristic finding is "scalloping" of the small bowel folds, which represent defects (bites) in the mucosa. Another "trick" is to fill the second–third portion of the duodenum with water. Water magnifies the endoscopic image. In normal cases, small villi will be easily seen swaying back and forth under water. If the villi are blunted, diminished, or absent, celiac disease should be suspected and biopsies should be obtained from the distal portion of the duodenum.

Dye enhancement techniques

Dye enhancement techniques may assist the recognition of inconspicuous mucosal lesions such as those found in celiac disease. Dye spraying (chromoscopy) is best achieved by spraying with a tube and fine nozzle applied close to the mucosa. The dye fills the interstices, highlighting irregularities in architecture. Indigo carmine is used most commonly. Intravital staining is an alternative approach to lesion enhancement. Stains such as methylene blue, Lugol's solution and toluidine blue may be taken up preferentially in diseased mucosa (such as intestinal metaplasia). Fluorescent stains (given intravenously) may highlight lesions under special conditions such as ultraviolet illumination. Optical techniques such as narrow band imaging (NBI), Fuji Intelligent Chromo Endoscopy (FICE) and iScan may offer similar benefit for identifying mucosal lesions without the need for dye.

Specimen collection

It is important to emphasize the need for close collaboration between endoscopy and laboratory staff. The diagnostic yield from endoscopic specimens will be maximized if laboratory staff are involved in defining the methods for specimen handling and transmission. Specimens should reach the laboratory with precise details of their origin and the specific clinical question that needs to be answered. Pathologists who routinely receive a copy of the endoscopy findings (and later follow-up) are more likely to give timely and relevant reports. Regular review sessions should be part of the quality improvement process.

Biopsy techniques

Biopsy specimens are taken with cupped forceps. The lesion should be approached face-on, so that firm and direct pressure can be applied to it with the widely opened cups. Pressure is easier to apply if the forceps are kept close to the endoscope tip. Better control is achieved by advancing the scope to the target rather than the forceps. Similarly, specimens from the esophagus are best taken by angling the tip of the endoscope acutely against the wall with the forceps barely protruding. The forceps are closed gently but firmly by an assistant and withdrawn. Forceps with a central spike make it easier to take specimens from lesions that have to be approached tangentially (e.g. in the esophagus). Spiked forceps may also allow for two specimens to be taken before withdrawing the forceps, as the spike acts to hold the first biopsy while the second is obtained. Some experts prefer not to use spiked forceps because of the risk of accidental skin puncture.

Ulcer biopsies should be taken from the ulcer rim in all four quadrants; basal specimens may be taken if a viral process is suspected, but for other entities they usually yield only slough. When sampling proliferative tumors it is wise to avoid necrotic areas, as they often produce nondiagnostic specimens.

The methods for handling and fixing specimens should be established after discussion with the relevant pathologist. Some prefer samples to be gently flattened on paper or other surfaces such as cellulose filter (Millipore, etc.). The cellulose filter method of biopsy mounting has considerable advantages for the management of multiple small endoscopic biopsies: they adhere well to the filter and are rarely lost; they are mounted in sequence so that errors of location are impossible; and they allow the histopathologist to view serial sections of six to eight biopsies at a time in a row across a single microscope slide. A 15-mm strip of cellulose filter (just less than the width of a glass slide) has a pencil-ruled or printed central line and a notch or mark made at one end (Fig 4.28a). Each biopsy is eased out of the forceps cup with the tip of a micropipette or toothpick (to avoid needle-stick injuries) (Fig 4.28b), placed exactly onto the line and patted flat (Fig 4.28c). The strip with its line of biopsies is placed into fixative (Fig 4.28d). In the laboratory it is processed, wax-mounted in the correct orientation (Fig 4.28e), sectioned through the line of biopsies on the filter (Fig 4.28f), positioned on

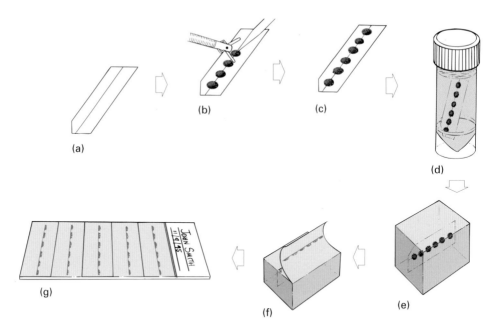

Fig 4.28 Stages in placing biopsies onto the filter then fixing, sectioning, and mounting the specimens.

the microscope slide (Fig 4.28g), and then stained and examined without handling the biopsies individually at any stage. A dissecting microscope or hand lens can be used to orientate mucosal specimens before fixation if information is required about the mucosal architecture (e.g. duodenal biopsies in malabsorption).

If detection of *H. pylori* infection is important, a biopsy specimen should be taken from the gastric antrum (if on proton pump inhibitor also from body or fundus). The specimen requisition should specifically state if *H. pylori* is suspected, as some pathology labs will not routinely do additional stains for *H. pylori* on gastric biopsies.

Biopsy sites often bleed trivially but sometimes sufficiently to obscure the lesion before adequate samples have been taken. If this is the case, the area should be washed with a jet of water or a 1:100,000 solution of epinephrine (adrenaline). Bleeding of clinical significance is exceptionally rare.

Cytology techniques

Cytology specimens are taken under direct vision with a sleeved brush (Fig 4.29), which is passed through the instrument channel. The head of the brush is advanced out of its sleeve and rubbed and rolled repeatedly across the surface of the lesion; a circumferential sweep of the margin and base of an ulcer is desirable. The brush is then pulled back into the sleeve and both are withdrawn together. The brush is protruded, wiped over two or three glass slides and then rapidly fixed before drying damages the cells. The precise method of preparation (in the unit or laboratory) should be determined by the cytologist. Brushes should not be reused. A trap (Fig 4.30)

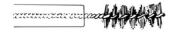

Fig 4.29 Cytology brush with outer sleeve.

can be used to collect cytology specimens. Suction through the channel after a biopsy procedure ("salvage cytology") also produces useful cellular material.

The value of brush cytology depends largely on the skill and enthusiasm of the cytopathologist. Many studies indicate that a combination of brush cytology and biopsy provides a higher yield than biopsy alone. In practice most endoscopists reserve cytology for lesions from which good biopsy specimens are difficult to obtain (e.g. tight esophageal strictures) and for resampling a suspicious lesion. They are also commonly used for collecting samples for suspected candida esophagitis. Taking aspiration samples for cytology though a needle may occasionally be useful.

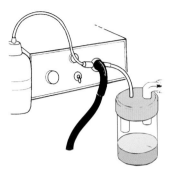

Fig 4.30 A suction trap to collect fluid specimens.

Sampling submucosal lesions

Standard biopsy specimens are usually normal in patients with submucosal lesions (such as benign tumors), as the forceps do not traverse the muscularis mucosae. One exception is in carcinoid tumors. These often originate from the deep mucosa and usually can be diagnosed from standard biopsy specimens. Larger and deeper specimens can be taken with a diathermy snare loop, as described with polypectomy in Chapter 7.

An alternative method for obtaining deeper tissue samples is to use a needle to obtain samples for cytology. EUS-guided fine needle aspiration is increasingly popular in this context.

Diagnostic endoscopy under special circumstances

Operated patients

Unless prevented by postoperative stenosis, endoscopy is the best method for diagnosis and exclusion of mucosal inflammation, recurrent ulcers, and tumors after upper gastrointestinal surgery. The endoscopist can document the size and arrangement of any outlet or anastomosis, but barium radiology and nuclear medicine techniques may be needed to give more information about motility and emptying disorders.

Experience is needed to appreciate the wide range of "normal" endoscopic appearance in the operated patient. Postoperative anatomy may be difficult to identify, particularly if there are multiple efferent lumens. Partial gastrectomy, gastroenterostomy, and pyloroplasty result in reflux of bile and intestinal juice. Resultant foaming in the stomach may obscure the endoscopic view and should be suppressed by flushing with a silicone suspension. Gastric distension is difficult to maintain in patients with a large gastric outlet; avoid pumping too much air and overdistending the intestine. Most patients who have undergone partial gastrectomy or gastroenterostomy have impressively hyperemic mucosae. Initially this is most marked close to the stoma, but atrophic gastritis is progressive, and plaques of grayish-white intestinal metaplasia may be seen. There is an increased risk of cancer in the gastric remnant, particularly close to the stoma. Cancers in this site can be difficult to recognize endoscopically. If the clinical suspicion for malignancy is high, multiple biopsy specimens from within 3 cm of the stoma should be taken.

Ulcers following partial gastrectomy or gastroenterostomy usually occur at or just beyond the anastomosis. Endoscopic diagnosis is usually simple, but the area just beneath the stoma may sometimes be difficult to survey completely using a forward-viewing instrument. A lateral-viewing endoscope may also sometimes allow a more complete survey in a scarred and tortuous pyloroplasty. Many surgeons use nonabsorbable sutures when performing an intestinal anastomosis. These can ulcerate through the mucosa and appear as black or green threads and loops. Their clinical significance remains controversial. Endoscopy is occasionally performed (for bleeding or stomal obstruction) within a few days of upper gastrointestinal tract surgery. In these cases air insufflation should be kept to a minimum.

Acute upper gastrointestinal bleeding

Bleeding provides special challenges for the endoscopist, and details are given in Chapter 5.

Endoscopy in children

Pediatric endoscopy is relatively simple with appropriate instruments and preparation; examination techniques are similar to those used in adults. The standard adult forward- and lateral-viewing instruments (8–11 mm diameter) can be used down to the age of about 2 years. Smaller pediatric instruments (5 mm diameter) may be needed in infants.

Endoscopy can be performed with little or no sedation in the first year of life. Fasted babies usually swallow the instrument avidly. Many endoscopists prefer to use general anesthesia beyond this age and into the mid-teens (especially for complex procedures), but some are satisfied with conscious sedation alone. This usually consists of a small dose of a benzodiazepine and generous doses of pethidine (Demerol). Even an apparently calm or well-sedated child may suddenly become briefly uncontrollable during intubation, and it is essential to swaddle the upper body and arms completely within a blanket before beginning, and to have an experienced nurse in charge of the biteguard (and suction). There is a risk of excessive air insufflation when using heavy sedation or anesthesia in the smallest children; it is wise to keep the abdomen exposed during examination and to palpate it regularly. Careful monitoring of oxygenation and the pulse is essential.

Endoscopy of the small intestine

Visualizing most or all of the small intestine is a challenge, but significant advances have been made in recent years. The third and fourth parts of the duodenum can usually be examined with standard forward-viewing endoscopes. This is often best achieved (as with colonoscopy) by pulling back to straighten the scope, deflating the stomach, applying abdominal pressure and maybe changing the patient's position.

Deep enteroscopy. Longer and more flexible endoscopes ("enteroscopes") can be pushed into the upper jejunum, but deeper insertion requires adjuvant devices. The simplest is a stiffening overtube, which prevents bowing in the stomach. Better results are now obtained with balloon-assisted enteroscopy and spiral enteroscopy. Enteroscopes with sleeves and one or two inflatable balloons allow skilled endoscopists to navigate large portions of the small bowel. The balloon acts as an intermittent "tether" as the scope is repeatedly straightened, then advanced. The same type of instrument can be used though the anus, to allow ileoscopy from below. Spiral enteroscopy involves a sleeve with a "corkscrew" device and has similar yield to balloon-assisted enteroscopy. Despite these developments, the extent of mucosal examination is variable and unpredictable. The procedure does cause some mucosal artifacts, which may mimic erosions.

Capsule endoscopy is a paradigm shift in digestive endoscopy, a remarkable technical achievement. Essentially the patient swallows a small camera (about the size of a Brazil nut), which transmits images to an external receiver. The images are examined at leisure. This technique has become popular for examining patients with gastrointestinal bleeding that is unexplained after standard procedures. Its use is being extended into screening the esophagus and even the colon. The capsule does not currently have any therapeutic potential, so lesions, when found, often must be sought again and treated by deep enteroscopy or surgery.

Further reading

American Society for Gastrointestinal Endoscopy. The role of endoscopy in the surveillance of premalignant conditions of the upper gastrointestinal tract. *Gastrointest Endosc* 2006; **63**:570–80.

Cohen J (ed.) *Advanced Digestive Endoscopy: Comprehensive Atlas of High Resolution Endoscopy and Narrowband Imaging.* Massachusettes: Blackwell Publishing Ltd, 2007.

Cotton PB, Sung J (eds) *Advanced Digestive Endoscopy ebook; Upper endoscopy.* Blackwell Publications, 2008. (available online at www.gastrohep.com).

Sidhu R, Sanders DS, Morris AJ, McAlindon ME. Guidelines on small bowel enteroscopy and capsule endoscopy in adults. *Gut* 2008; **57**: 125–36.

Atlas of Gastrointestinal Endoscopy, 4th Edition. Yamada T, Willingham F, Brugge WR, 2009. Blackwell Publishing Ltd www.endoatlas.com;

Willingham FF, Brugge WR. Upper Gastrointestinal Endoscopy. In: Yamada T (ed.) *Atlas of Gastroenterology,* 4th Edition. Oxford: Wiley-Blackwell, 2009. (available online at http://onlinelibrary.wiley.com/doi/10.1002/9781444303414.ch85/summary).

Chapter video clips

Video 4.1 Endoscopic view of direct vision insertion

Video 4.2 Full insertion and examination

Now check your understanding—go to

www.wiley.com/go/cottonwilliams/practicalgastroenterology

CHAPTER 5

Therapeutic Upper Endoscopy

Today's gastroenterologists have a major role in the interventional treatment of many upper gastrointestinal problems. Established techniques include the management of dysphagia (due to benign and malignant esophageal stenoses and achalasia), polyps, gastric and duodenal stenoses, foreign bodies, acute bleeding, and nutritional support. Other innovative therapies, such as the endoscopic treatment of reflux, and of obesity, are being developed.

Benign esophageal strictures

Gastroesophageal reflux is the commonest cause of benign esophageal strictures. Other causes include specific esophageal inflammations and infections, medications, caustic ingestion, extrinsic compression, and therapeutic interventions (surgery, endoscopy, and radiation).

In general, dysphagia occurs when the esophageal lumen is less than about 13 mm. It follows that easy passage of a standard endoscope (8–10 mm diameter) does not exclude a problem, or the possible need for treatment.

Dilation methods

Dilation is used only as part of an overall treatment plan, with due attention also to diet, lifestyle modification, and necessary medications. Surgery is needed in a few recalcitrant cases.

Even though there are many dilation techniques and varieties of equipment, they fall into two main categories: *mechanical* (push-type or bougie) or *balloon* dilators. While the exact mechanism is not clear, the mechanical dilators exert a longitudinal and radial force, dilating proximal to distal on the stricture, opposed to the purely radial force delivered simultaneously across the stricture by the balloon dilators.

Mild strictures can be treated simply in some patients with mercury-weighted dilators (such as Maloney bougies) without sedation. Dilating balloons or graduated bougies are used when the stenosis is tight or tortuous, under endoscopic and/or fluoroscopic control (over a guidewire), to ensure correct placement. Both methods are effective and their relative merits are debated. Bougie techniques give a better "feel" of the stricture, which may be an important safety factor.

Cotton and Williams' Practical Gastrointestinal Endoscopy: The Fundamentals, Seventh Edition.
Adam Haycock, Jonathan Cohen, Brian P Saunders, Peter B Cotton, and Christopher B Williams.
© 2014 John Wiley & Sons, Ltd. Published 2014 by John Wiley & Sons, Ltd.
Companion Website: www.wiley.com/go/cottonwilliams/practicalgastroenterology

Certain strictures, particularly those due to irradiation or cor-
rosive ingestion, are more difficult to dilate. Procedures may need
to be repeated several times with gradual increase in dilator size—
too rapid an increase can result in perforation. As a general rule,
no more than three dilators of progressively increasing size should
be used during a single session.

Dilation can provoke bacteremia, so antibiotic prophylaxis
against endocarditis should be considered in patients with significant cardiac lesions (see Table 3.1).

Balloon dilation

Balloons are designed to be passed through the endoscope channel,
often with a guidewire (Fig 5.1). They range from 3 to 8 cm in
length and from 6 to 40 mm in diameter (some multidiameter with
increasing pressures). Most strictures are short, but medium-length
balloons (about 5 cm) are convenient to use, as they are less likely
to "pop out" of the stricture than shorter ones. Lubrication makes
insertion easier, either applied directly to the balloon with a silicone
spray or by injecting 1–2 mL silicone oil down the endoscope
channel followed by 10 mL air. The stricture is examined endoscopically, and its diameter is assessed. Tight strictures should be
approached initially with small balloons, typically corresponding to
the diameter of the stricture. The guidewire and soft tip of an
appropriately sized balloon is passed gently through the stricture
under direct vision. The balloons are fairly translucent, so that it is
usually possible to observe the "waist" endoscopically during the
procedure and to judge the effect. Balloons are distended with
water (or contrast medium) to the pressure(s) recommended by
the manufacturer conventionally for 1–2 minutes, though as little
as 30 seconds may be sufficient.

The "through-the-scope" (TTS) balloon dilation technique
has several advantages. It can be performed as part of the initial
endoscopy, and does not normally require fluoroscopic monitoring.
The results should be obvious immediately, and the endoscope
can be passed through the stricture to complete the endoscopic
examination.

Bougie dilation

Dilation can be performed with graduated bougies that are passed
over a guidewire. This ensures that the dilator will pass correctly
through the stricture (and not into a diverticulum or necrotic
tumor, or through the wall of a hiatus hernia). This security exists
only if the position of the wire is checked frequently using fluoroscopy or a fixed external landmark. Fluoroscopic monitoring is
essential when tight and complex strictures are being treated.

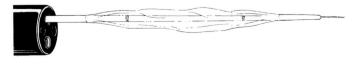

Fig 5.1 A deflated "through-the-scope" (TTS) balloon dilator and guidewire.

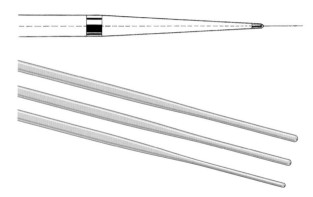

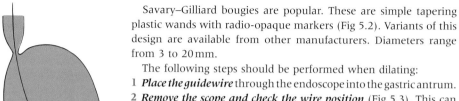

Fig 5.2 Tips of Savary-Gilliard (above) and American Endoscopy (below) dilators for use over a guidewire.

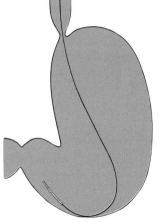

Fig 5.3 A dilator guidewire positioned in the gastric antrum.

Savary–Gilliard bougies are popular. These are simple tapering plastic wands with radio-opaque markers (Fig 5.2). Variants of this design are available from other manufacturers. Diameters range from 3 to 20 mm.

The following steps should be performed when dilating:

1 *Place the guidewire* through the endoscope into the gastric antrum.
2 *Remove the scope and check the wire position* (Fig 5.3). This can be done fluoroscopically, or by checking the length of wire outside the patient. If the guidewire has distance markers, keep the 60 cm mark close to the teeth.
3 *Choose a bougie* that will pass relatively easily through the stricture and slide it over the guidewire down close to the mouth. Lubricate the tip of the bougie.
4 *Hold the bougie shaft in the left hand and push it in*, simultaneously applying countertraction on the guidewire with the right hand. Keep the left elbow extended so that the dilator cannot travel too far when resistance "gives" (Fig 5.4). This reduces the chance of advancing too rapidly.
5 *Increase the size of the bougies* progressively, checking the guidewire position repeatedly, but observe the rule of three, i.e. do not use more than three sizes above the size at which significant resistance is first felt.
6 *After dilation, check the effect endoscopically*. Take biopsy and cytology samples if necessary.

Refractory strictures

For some patients, an intensive dilation schedule and maximal gastroesophageal reflux therapy is not adequate to provide symptomatic relief. Several alternative endoscopic techniques have been used for such recalcitrant strictures.

• *Corticosteroid injection.* The injection of corticosteroids into a stricture is believed to reduce scar formation by preventing collagen deposition and enhancing local breakdown. Before stricture dilation, a standard sclerotherapy injection needle is used to deliver 0.2 mL triamcinolone acetonide into each of the four quadrants of the narrowest area of the stricture. The evidence base for this

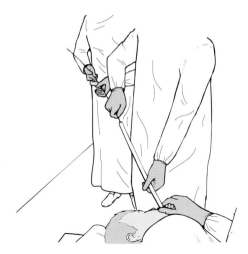

Fig 5.4 Advance the dilator with the left hand and the elbow extended to avoid sudden overinsertion. Keep traction on the wire with the right hand.

practice is limited, and small studies have not shown it to be effective in strictures secondary to inflammatory bowel disease.

• *Nonmetal stents.* Removable nonmetal stents have recently been introduced as an alternative for refractory strictures. Covered self-expanding plastic stents can be effective for benign strictures in the short term, but complications of stent migration and chest pain are common and limit overall clinical success. Biodegradable stents can also be effective in the short term (90 days) but also have high complication rates, and sequential stenting may be required to maintain clinical efficacy.

Post-dilation management

Patients should be kept nil by mouth and under observation for at least 1 hour after dilation. Any complaint of pain should be taken seriously. Chest films and a water-soluble contrast swallow should be performed if there is any suspicion of perforation (perforation is discussed in detail under "Esophageal cancer palliation" below). A trial drink of water is given if progress has been satisfactory. The patient is then discharged with instructions to keep to a soft diet overnight, plus appropriate medications and a follow-up plan. Studies have shown that the use of proton pump inhibitors (PPIs) in patients with benign peptic strictures reduces the need for subsequent dilation when compared with H_2 antagonists and should therefore be added after the procedure. Dilation can be repeated within a few days in severe cases, and then subsequently every few weeks until swallowing has been fully restored.

Achalasia

Manometry provides the "gold standard" for the diagnosis of achalasia, but endoscopy is also essential to exclude submucosal or fundal

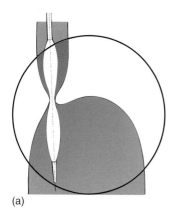

(a)

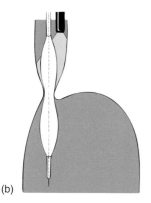

(b)

Fig 5.5 Achalasia dilating balloons (before full inflation). (a) Checked fluoroscopically. (b) Visualized endoscopically.

malignancy. Achalasia can be treated with surgical or laparoscopic myotomy, balloon dilation, or with injections of botulinum toxin.

Balloon dilation

Patients with achalasia often have food residue in the esophagus. They should take only a clear liquid diet for several days before the procedure, and large-bore tube lavage may be needed beforehand.

Many different techniques and balloons have been used. The balloon position can be checked radiologically, or under direct vision with the endoscope alongside the balloon shaft (Fig 5.5), or even by a retroversion maneuver with the balloon fitted over the endoscope shaft. We prefer to place a guidewire endoscopically, identify the lower esophageal sphincter fluoroscopically, and then dilate with a balloon under fluoroscopic control.

Achalasia balloons are available with diameters of 30, 35, and 40 mm. It is wise to start with the smallest balloon, warning the patient that repeat treatments may be necessary if symptoms persist or recur quickly.

Inflation is maintained at the recommended pressure for up to 1 minute, and may be repeated. Observe the waist on the balloon fluoroscopically: inadequate expansion may indicate other pathology. Conversely, abrupt disappearance of the waist may suggest perforation (perforation is discussed under "Esophageal cancer palliation" below).

There is usually some blood on the balloon after the procedure. Close observation is mandatory for at least 4 hours. Chest radiographs and a water-soluble contrast swallow are done routinely in some units. Nothing should be given by mouth until the patient and the radiographs have been examined by the endoscopist personally. A trial drink of water is given under supervision. The uncomplicated patient can return to a normal diet on the next day.

Botulinum toxin

Treatment with botulinum toxin can be applied by direct free-hand endoscopic injection into the area of the lower esophageal sphincter, or using endoscopic ultrasound guidance. Reported results are good but short-lived, and the majority of patients require multiple procedures to maintain clinical efficacy. The value of this method may therefore be limited to individuals in whom other procedures are unacceptable or contraindicated.

Esophageal cancer palliation

Barium studies and endoscopy have complementary roles in assessing the site and nature of esophageal neoplasms. Endoscopic ultrasonography is the most accurate staging tool. Endoscopic management can help to improve swallowing in the majority of patients who are unsuitable for surgery because of intercurrent disease or tumor extent. However, endoscopists should be aware of their treatment limitations and should balance technological enthusiasm with full consideration of the patient's quality of life (and likely duration of survival). Achieving a large lumen will not restore normal swallowing. The goal should be to achieve adequate swallowing at the lowest risk and inconvenience to the patient.

Palliative techniques

Several methods can be used to palliate malignant dysphagia. The abrupt onset of severe dysphagia may be due to the impaction of a food bolus, which can be removed endoscopically by standard techniques. Malignant strictures can be dilated using wire-guided balloons or bougies, taking great care not to split the tumor by being overambitious. The bulk of an exophytic tumor can be reduced by various ablation techniques. Monopolar diathermy is readily available, but it is difficult to control the depth of injury, and charring occurs quickly. Local injection of a toxic agent such as absolute alcohol is also effective, if somewhat unpredictable. Laser ablation (using the Nd:YAG laser) was popular in previous years, largely because a "no-touch" technique seemed esthetically preferable, but the equipment is expensive, and similar results can be achieved using argon plasma coagulation (APC), which is simpler and cheaper. It also has the advantage that the energy can be applied tangentially.

   Ablative techniques are most useful in short exophytic lesions, and for recurrences after surgery or stenting. All of the methods are somewhat hazardous (perforation rate up to 5%) and are rarely effective for more than a few weeks. As a result, there is an increasing tendency to place stents as a primary measure. Chemotherapy, radiotherapy, and photodynamic therapy are also used.

Esophageal stenting

There are good indications for using esophageal stents, but insertion can be very challenging, and is not to be undertaken lightly by the endoscopist or patient. The best candidates are mid-esophageal tumors in patients with a prognosis limited to weeks or months, and in those with tracheoesophageal fistulae. Stents cannot be used when the tumor extends to within 2 cm of the cricopharyngeus. They may also function less well in lesions at the cardia because of the angulation, and reflux may be a problem. Newer stents with an antireflux mechanism may theoretically reduce this complication.

   Great care must be taken when dysphagia is caused by very large tumors, as stent placement may compromise the airway. Prior bronchoscopy is appropriate in such cases, and trial inflation of a balloon may indicate what diameter is tolerable.

Stent variety

Traditional plastic stents with fixed diameters have largely been replaced by self-expandable metal or plastic stents (SEMS and SEPS, respectively), as they are easier and less hazardous to insert. Many types of **SEMS** are now available. They vary according to the type, diameter, and weave of the wires (which determine their expansile strength), their shapes and sizes, and the presence or absence of a covering membrane (Fig 5.6). This membrane is helpful in patients with fistulae, and reduces tumor ingrowth, but some mesh must be left exposed to prevent migration. Stents for

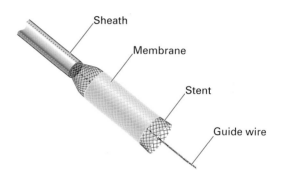

Fig 5.6 Covered metal mesh stent.

use in the esophagus have luminal diameters of 15–24 mm, and lengths of 6–15 cm. They are compressed into delivery systems of 6–11 mm. Most expand gradually over a few days, and become fully incorporated in the esophageal wall so that they cannot be removed. Less powerful stents—although easy to place and well tolerated—may not expand sufficiently to relieve the patient's symptoms, even with balloon dilation.

Newer **SEPS** are similar to SEMS in concept. The main advantage over metal stents is the ability to be repositioned or removed. Disadvantages include a larger, more difficult delivery system and higher migration rate. Currently, SEPS are indicated for benign esophageal diseases.

Stent insertion

Before insertion the patient should be fully informed about the aims of the procedure, the potential serious risks, and the (few) alternatives. Antibiotic prophylaxis should be considered. The lesion is assessed carefully by radiology and endoscopy, and bougie dilation is performed if necessary (to about 12 mm) to allow passage of the endoscope if possible. The upper and lower margins of the tumor are marked by endoscopic injection of contrast medium using a sclerotherapy needle. A guidewire is placed, and its position checked by fluoroscopy.

The stent system is then introduced over the guidewire and the stent is released by gradual withdrawal of the sleeve. Correct positioning of the stent is judged fluoroscopically (using the contrast medium marks), and then by repeat endoscopy.

Post-stent management

Patients are usually kept in the hospital overnight under observation because of the immediate risk of perforation and bleeding, and for necessary pain control. Chest and water-soluble contrast swallow radiographic studies are performed after about 2 hours. Clear fluids can be given after 4 hours if there have been no adverse developments.

Patients must understand the limitations of the stent, and the need to maintain a soft diet with plenty of fluids during and after

meals. Written instructions should be provided and relatives counseled. Overambitious eating or inadequate chewing may result in
obstruction. If food impaction occurs, the bolus can usually be
removed or fragmented endoscopically using snares, biopsy forceps,
or balloons.

Stent dysfunction due to tumor overgrowth can be managed by
endoscopic ablation or placement of another stent inside the first.
SEPS offer the option of removal. Gastroesophageal reflux can be
a problem with stents crossing the cardia. Patients may need to
sleep propped up, and to use acid-reducing medications. Occasionally, a good result from chemotherapy or radiotherapy may make
it possible to remove a stent. For the same reason, stents (especially
the covered variety) may migrate spontaneously. Recovery of
stents from the stomach can be challenging.

Esophageal perforation

The endoscopic treatment of esophageal strictures is relatively safe
in most cases using optimal techniques. Perforations do occur,
however, especially with complex and malignant strictures
approached by inexperienced or overconfident endoscopists. The
rate is approximately 0.1% in benign esophageal strictures, 1% in
achalasia dilation, and 5–10% in treatment of malignant lesions.
The risk is minimized by taking the process step by step—gradually
and deliberately. Never try to dilate to the largest balloon or bougie
simply because it is available.

Early suspicion and recognition of perforation is the key to successful management, and no complaint should be ignored. The
problem is usually obvious clinically; the patient is distressed and
in pain. Signs of subcutaneous emphysema may develop within a
few hours. Radiographic studies should be performed. Surgical
consultation is mandatory when perforation is seriously suspected
or confirmed. Many confined perforations have been managed
conservatively, with nil oral intake, intravenous (IV) fluids, and
antibiotics—with or without placement of a sump tube across the
perforation.

The choice between surgical and conservative management (and
the timing of surgical intervention if conservative management
appears to be failing) is often difficult; review of the literature
shows varied and strong opinions. Conservative management is
more likely to be appropriate when the perforation is in the neck;
because the mediastinum is not contaminated, local surgical drainage can be performed simply when necessary. Perforation through
a tumor can be treated immediately with a covered stent if the
lumen can be found and if surgical cure is not possible.

Gastric and duodenal stenoses

Functionally significant stenoses may occur in the stomach or duodenum as a result of disease (tumors and ulcers) and following
surgical intervention (e.g. hiatus hernia repair, gastroenterostomy,
pyloroplasty, and gastroplasty). Balloon dilation of stenosed surgical

stomas is usually effective (except in the case of banded gastroplasty with a rigid silicone ring). Pyloroduodenal stenosis caused by ulceration can be relieved by balloon dilation, but recurrence is common. Expandable stents are being used with remarkably good effect in patients with malignant stenosis of the stomach and duodenum.

Gastric and duodenal polyps and tumors

Endoscopic polypectomy is frequently used in the colon, and many of the techniques (see Chapter 7) can be applied in the stomach and duodenum. Polyps are much less common in the stomach and duodenum than in the colon, and are rare in the esophagus. Many of these polyps are sessile, and some are largely submucosal, making endoscopic treatment more difficult and hazardous. The possibility of a transmural lesion should be considered, and endoscopic ultrasonography may be helpful in making a treatment decision; surgical (or laparoscopic) resection may be safer. Injecting the base of sessile gastric and duodenal polyps with epinephrine (adrenaline; 1 : 10,000) may make removal easier, and may reduce the risk of bleeding. Some endoscopists use detachable loops for the same purpose.

Endoscopic mucosal resection (EMR) has been developed in Japan for removal of sessile lesions up to 2 cm or more in diameter. The lesion is raised up by injecting a cushion of saline/epinephrine, and then sucked into a special transparent plastic cap attached to the tip of the endoscope. The lesion is then resected with a snare loop incorporated in the cap (Fig 5.7).

Snare diathermy techniques can be used also to obtain large biopsy specimens when the gastric mucosa appears thickened, and when standard biopsy techniques have failed to provide a diagnosis.

Gastric polypectomy, EMR, and snare loop biopsy techniques can cause bleeding and perforation. They also leave an ulcer; it is wise to prescribe acid-suppressant medication for a few weeks.

Foreign bodies

Foreign bodies are mainly a problem in children, in elderly patients with poor teeth, and in the drunk or deranged. The problem is obvious if the patient suddenly cannot swallow, and especially if a missing object is visible on a radiograph. However, many instances are less straightforward. Patients may not know that they have swallowed a foreign object. Some common items (e.g. bones and drink-can tags) are not radiopaque. It is therefore necessary to maintain a high index of suspicion.

Chest and abdominal radiographs (with lateral views) are appropriate, as they may identify radiopaque objects or signs of esophageal perforation such as mediastinal or subcutaneous air. A water-soluble contrast swallow examination is helpful in some patients, but it is not necessary, and is potentially hazardous if dysphagia is complete.

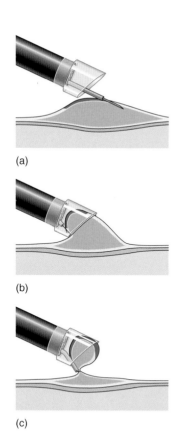

(a)

(b)

(c)

Fig 5.7 Endoscopic mucosal resection. (a) Inject a saline cushion below the lesion. (b) Suck the lesion into the transparent cap. (c) Snare and resect the lesion.

Many foreign bodies pass spontaneously, but active treatment should be initiated within hours in some circumstances.

Urgent treatment is required for:
- patients who cannot swallow saliva
- impacted sharp objects
- ingestion of button batteries (which can disintegrate and cause local damage).

Foreign body extraction

Objects impacted at or above the cricopharyngeus are usually best removed by surgeons with rigid instruments. Flexible endoscopy now takes precedence in most (but not all) other situations. The use of an overtube increases the therapeutic options (Fig 5.8). Endoscopy can usually be accomplished with conscious sedation, but general anesthesia should be considered in children and uncooperative adults, and when there is concern about the airway.

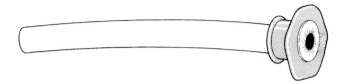

Fig 5.8 An overtube with biteguard.

Food impaction

An IV injection of glucagon (0.5–1.0 mg) may help to release a food impaction by relaxing the esophagus. The use of meat tenderizer is discouraged, as severe pulmonary complications have resulted. Meat can be removed as a single piece endoscopically, using a polypectomy snare, tri-prong grasper, or retrieval basket. Another approach is to use strong suction on the end of an overtube or a banding sleeve. Take care not to lose the bolus near the larynx. Food that has been impacted for several hours can usually be broken up (e.g. with a snare), and the pieces pushed into the stomach. This must be done carefully, especially if there is any question of a bone being present.

Most patients with impacted food have some esophageal narrowing (due to a benign reflux stricture or Schatzki ring). The endoscopist's task is not complete until this has been checked and treated. Sometimes it is possible to maneuver a small endoscope past the food bolus and to use the tip to dilate the distal stricture; the food can then be pushed through the narrowed area. Usually, dilation can be performed at the time of food extraction, but it should be delayed if there is substantial edema or ulceration, or concern for eosinophilic esophagitis, as this condition increases the risk of esophageal perforation.

Gastric bezoars

Gastric bezoars are aggregations of fibrous animal or vegetable material. They are usually found in association with delayed gastric emptying (e.g. postoperative stenosis or dysfunction). Most masses can be fragmented with biopsy forceps or a polypectomy snare, but more distal bolus obstruction may result if fragmentation is inadequate. Various enzyme preparations (e.g. cellulase) have been recommended to facilitate disruption, but these are rarely necessary or effective. Large gastric bezoars are best disrupted and removed by inserting a large-bore lavage tube, and instilling and removing 2–3 L tap water with a large syringe. Other techniques have included infusion of a carbonated drink, mechanical or electrohydraulic or extracorporeal lithotripsy. The cause of gastric-emptying dysfunction should be evaluated, and treated.

Swallowed objects

The range of swallowed objects is amazing. Foreign bodies trapped in the esophagus should always be removed. Sharp objects (such as open safety pins) are best withdrawn into the tip of an overtube (Fig 5.9); sometimes it is safer to use a rigid esophagoscope.

Most objects that reach the stomach will pass spontaneously, but there are exceptions that demand early intervention:
• sharp and pointed objects have a 15–20% chance of causing perforation (usually at the ileo-cecal valve), and should be extracted while still in the stomach or proximal duodenum
• objects >2 cm diameter and longer than 5 cm are unlikely to pass from the stomach spontaneously and should be removed if possible.

Button batteries usually pass spontaneously when they have reached the stomach; a purgative should be given to accelerate the process. Those that do not pass into the stomach and remain in the esophagus should be removed promptly as contact with the esophageal wall can quickly lead to necrosis and perforation.

Foreign bodies rarely pass out of the stomach in children who have had pyloromyotomies.

Endoscopists should resist the temptation to attempt removal of condoms containing cocaine or other hard drugs, as rupture can lead to a massive overdose. Asymptomatic patients can be managed expectantly until the packet passes. Use of polyethylene glycol lavage solutions are safe and likely accelerate the rate of clearance. For individuals with obstruction or perforation or narcotic toxicity without an antidote (e.g. cocaine) immediate surgical evaluation and removal are the safest option.

Golden rules for foreign body removal:
• be sure that your extraction procedure is really necessary
• think before you start, and rehearse outside the patient
• do not make the situation worse
• do not be slow to get surgical or anesthetic assistance
• protect the esophagus, pharynx, and bronchial tree during withdrawal (with an overtube or endotracheal anesthesia)
• remove sharp objects with the point trailing.

Extraction devices

The endoscopist should have several specialized tools available, in addition to the overtube. There are forceps with claws or flat blades

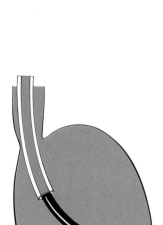

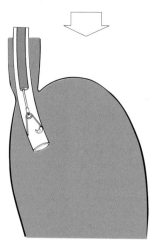

Fig 5.9 Remove sharp foreign bodies with a protecting overtube.

designed to grasp coins (Fig 5.10); a tri-prong extractor is useful for meat (Fig 5.11). Many objects can be grasped with a polypectomy snare or stone-retrieval basket. Others can be collected in a retrieval net. A protector hood can be placed at the tip of the endoscope to protect the esophageal and pharyngeal wall from sharp edges of the foreign body during extraction. Any object with a hole (such as a key or ring) can be removed by passing a thread through the hole. The endoscope is passed into the stomach with biopsy forceps or a snare closed within its tip, grasping a thread, which passes down the outside of the instrument (Fig 5.12). The forceps are advanced and the thread passed through the object, dropped and retrieved from the other side.

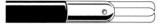

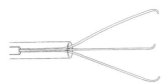

Fig 5.10 Foreign-body extraction forceps.

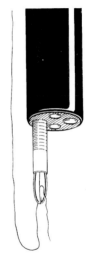

Acute bleeding

Acute upper gastrointestinal bleeding (hematemesis and/or melena) is a common medical problem for which endoscopy has become the primary diagnostic and therapeutic technique. Emergency endoscopy is a challenging task. There is considerable potential for benefit, but also for risk. These techniques require experience, nerve, and judgment. Safety considerations are paramount. The endoscopist should be well trained, working with familiar equipment and expert nurses. Unstable patients should be under supervision in an intensive care environment. Sedation should be given cautiously, and precautions taken to avoid pulmonary aspiration. Patients with severe bleeding are often best examined under general anesthesia, with the airway protected by a cuffed endotracheal tube.

Many different endoscopic techniques have been developed. These include injection with saline/epinephrine or sclerosant or fibrin, banding, thermal probes (heat probe, bipolar, or monopolar electrocoagulation, APC, and lasers), and clipping. Endoscopic suturing will soon be added to this list. Many trials have compared different techniques, but the experience of the endoscopist—and familiarity with a particular technique—is probably the most important determinant of success. Laser photocoagulation initially became popular because it was assumed that it was safer not to touch the lesion. It has become clear, however, that direct pressure with some probes (and injection treatment) provides an important tamponade and "coaptation" effect (see Fig 5.18), and increases the size of vessel that can be treated.

The *timing* of endoscopy is important. Examination can be delayed to a convenient time (e.g. the next morning) in patients who appear to be stable, but the endoscopic team must be prepared to go into action within hours (after immediate resuscitation) in certain circumstances. Several validated systems exist to risk stratify patients for endoscopy, including the Rockall Score and the Glasgow–Blatchford Score (see Tables 5.1 and 5.2).

Fig 5.11 A triprong grasping device.

Fig 5.12 Take a thread down with the forceps to pass through any object with a hole in it, such as a ring or key.

Table 5.1 Rockall Score

	0	1	2	3
Age (years)	<60	60–79	>79	–
Degree of shock	Systolic BP >100 mmHg Heart rate <100/min	Systolic BP >100 mmHg Heart rate >100/min	Systolic BP <100 mmHg Heart rate >100/min	–
Comorbidities	None	–	Heart failure Ischaemic heart disease	Renal/liver failure Disseminated cancer
Endoscopic diagnosis	Mallory–Weiss tear No lesion	All other diagnosis	Upper GI malignancy	–
Stigmata of bleeding	None or dark spot only	–	Visible/spurting vessel, blood, clot	–

Table 5.2 Glasgow–Blatchford Score

(a) Blood urea (mmol/L)	Score	(c) Systolic BP (mmHg)	Score
≥6.5 <8.0	2	100–109	1
≥8.0 <10.0	3	90–99	2
≥10.0 <25	4	<90	3
≥25	6	**(d) Other markers**	
(b1) Haemoglobin for men (g/dL)		Pulse ≥ 100 beats/min	1
≥12.0 <13.0	1	Presentation with malaena	1
≥10.0 <12.0	3	Presentation with syncope	2
<10.0	6	Hepatic disease	2
(b2) Haemoglobin for women (g/dL)		Cardiac failure	2
≥10.0 <12.0	1		
<10.0	6		

Indications for emergency endoscopy include:
- continued active bleeding requiring intervention
- suspicion of variceal bleeding
- presence of an aortic graft
- severe rectal bleeding with inconclusive colonic studies
- elderly patients with cardiovascular compromise on presentation.

Lavage?

Blood clots may obscure the view in the stomach and duodenum. Standard gastric lavage is rarely effective, even when performed personally with a large-bore tube. Endoscopes with a large channel (or two channels) allow better flushing and suction. An alternative

approach is to start the procedure with an overtube over the endoscope (Fig 5.13). If blood is encountered, the endoscope can be
removed and blood clots sucked directly through the overtube;
lavage can be performed.

A diagnosis can usually be made even if the stomach cannot be
emptied completely. Lesions are rare on the greater curvature,
where the blood pools in the standard left lateral position. Changing the patient's position somewhat should improve the survey, but
turning completely on the right side is hazardous unless the airway
is protected.

An alternative to lavage may be the use of pharmacologic agents,
such as metoclopramide or erythromycin, to accelerate gastric
emptying. Studies have shown that a single dose of IV erythromycin prior to endoscopy can significantly improve visibility and
reduce the need for second-look endoscopy.

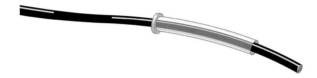

Fig 5.13 Overtube with endoscope.

Bleeding lesions

Lesions that cause acute bleeding are well known. Endoscopy has
highlighted the fact that many patients are found to have more
than one mucosal lesion (e.g. esophageal varices and acute gastric
erosions). Thus, a complete examination of the esophagus, stomach,
and duodenum should be performed in every bleeding patient, no
matter what is seen en route. A lesion should be incriminated as
the bleeding source only if it is actively bleeding at the time of
endoscopy, or shows characteristic stigmata, for example, an ulcer
with adherent clot or a visible vessel. If the patient has presented
with hematemesis, and complete upper endoscopy shows only a
single lesion (even without any of these features), it is likely to be
the bleeding source. This is not necessarily the case if the presentation has been with melena, or if the examination takes place more
than 48 hours after bleeding, since acute lesions such as mucosal
tears and erosions may already have healed. Likewise, varices
cannot be incriminated definitely unless they are bleeding or show
specific stigmata.

Variceal treatments

Endoscopic treatment of esophageal (and gastric) varices can be
helpful in patients who are bleeding, or who have recently bled.
Prophylactic treatment remains controversial. Intervention in the
presence of active bleeding is challenging. Patients are often very
sick, and the views may be poor. It may be helpful to tilt the patient
slightly head up, or to apply traction on a gastric balloon to reduce

the flow of blood. Often it is wise to defer endoscopy for several hours, pending the effect of pharmacological treatment. Sengstaten–Blakemore tube tamponade or transjugular intrahepatic portosystemic shunt (TIPS) treatments may be appropriate.

Elimination of varices usually involves a series of treatments. Endoscopic management should be seen as only part of a patient's overall care. Available techniques include banding, injection sclerosis, and combination techniques. Clips and loops have also been used recently.

Variceal banding

Banding is now considered the procedure of choice because it causes fewer ulcers and strictures than sclerotherapy and has a proven mortality benefit. Commercially available devices consist of a friction-fit sleeve for the endoscope tip, an inner cylinder preloaded with elastic bands, and a trip wire that passes up the endoscope channel (Fig. 5.14). The varix is sucked into the sleeve, and the band released by pulling on the wire. Multiple bands are applied in an upwards spiral fashion every 1–2 cm.

Banding can also be applied to gastric varices and to small ulcers (e.g. Dieulafoy lesions). Disadvantages to the band ligator include obscured visibility by blood during active bleeding and poor maneuverability, especially back into the stomach by the endoscope after band deployment.

Injection sclerotherapy

Injection sclerotherapy has been used for decades and is still the treatment of choice for gastric varices. Many adjuvant devices have been described, including overtubes with a lateral window and the use of balloons, either in the stomach to compress distal varices or on the scope itself to permit tamponade if bleeding occurs. However, most experts use a simple "free-hand" method, with a standard large-channel endoscope and a flexible, retractable needle (Fig. 5.15). Injections are given directly into the varices, starting close to the cardia (and below any bleeding site) and working spirally upwards for about 5 cm. Each injection consists of 1–2 mL of sclerosant, to a total of 20–40 mL.

Precise placement of the needle within the varix (as guided by co-injection of a dye such as methylene blue or by simultaneous manometric or radiographic techniques) may improve the results and reduce the complications. However, some experts believe that paravariceal injections are also effective, and it is often difficult to tell which has been achieved. If bleeding occurs on removal of the needle, it is usually helpful to tamponade the area simply by passing the endoscope into the stomach. The esophagogastric junction can be compressed directly if the endoscope is retroflexed.

Sclerosants

Several chemical agents are available as sclerosants. Sodium morrhuate (5%) and sodium tetradecylsulfate (STD) (1–1.5%) are

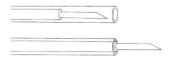

Fig 5.14 A retractable sclerotherapy needle.

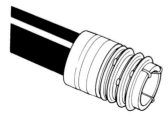

Fig 5.15 An esophageal banding device.

popular in the USA. Polidocanol (1%), ethanolamine oleate (5%), and STD are widely used in Europe. Efficacy, ulcerogenicity and the risk of complications run together, since it is the process of damage and healing by fibrosis that eradicates or buries the communicating veins, but may also cause stricturing. Endoscopic polymer injection is another alternative. The two cyanoacrylate agents most commonly used are not available in the USA. These polymers solidify almost immediately on contact with aqueous material. The endoscopist and nurse must use them carefully to provide an effective injection without gluing up the endoscope. Results are excellent, especially in gastric varices (which do not respond well to standard sclerotherapy). Many use this technique also in patients who relapse quickly after banding or sclerotherapy in the acute situation. Fibrin glue is an alternative which is now routinely used for treatment of gastric varices.

Care after variceal treatments

The risks of variceal treatment include all of the complications of emergency endoscopy (especially pulmonary aspiration).

Patients often have transient chest pain, odynophagia (pain on swallowing), and dysphagia. They should maintain a soft diet for a few days, avoid any medications that may irritate or cause bleeding, and take acid-suppressing agents. Treatment should be repeated in about a week in the context of acute bleeding, but should be delayed for several weeks when elective, to allow the lesions to heal. Delayed complications include esophageal stricturing, which is more common after sclerotherapy. Strictures can be dilated gingerly with standard methods.

Treatment of bleeding ulcers

Duodenal and gastric ulcers are still common causes of acute bleeding. About 80% will stop bleeding spontaneously. It is important, if possible, to predict those patients likely to rebleed and to select them for endoscopic treatment. We are guided by the size of the initial bleed, the overall status of the patient, and by the presence or absence of stigmata.

Ulcer stigmata

The following stigmata provide useful pointers when considering treatment options:
• *Active "spurters"* continue to bleed (or rebleed soon) in 70–80% of cases.
• *Ulcers with a "visible vessel"* have about a 50% chance of rebleeding.
• *Ulcers with an "adherent clot"* have about a 25–30% chance of rebleeding.
• *Clean ulcers do not rebleed*.

An important question is whether it is appropriate to wash clots off the base of an ulcer simply to check for these stigmata. Most endoscopists will do so in high-risk patients provided they are poised for treatment.

Fig 5.16 Teflon-coated tip of a heat probe with a water-jet opening.

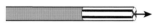

Fig 5.17 The tip of a multipolar probe with a central water jet.

Treatment modalities

The most popular hemostatic methods currently are injection, heat probe, bipolar probe, and combinations. Clips and other mechanical closure devices are being used increasingly and may be as efficacious when used alone as the other modalities are in combination.

• *Injection treatment*. Epinephrine in saline (1:10,000) is applied with a sclerotherapy needle in 0.5–1.0 mL aliquots around the base of the bleeding site, up to a total of 10 mL. Some prefer to use absolute alcohol in much smaller volumes (1–2 mL in 0.1 mL aliquots) or combinations of epinephrine with alcohol, or with the sclerosants used for the treatment of varices.

• The *heat probe* (Fig. 5.16) provides a constant temperature of 250°C. First tamponade, then apply several pulses of 30 J.

• The *bipolar (or multipolar) probe* (Fig. 5.17) provides bipolar electrocoagulation, which is assumed to be safer than monopolar diathermy (which produces an unpredictable depth of damage). Use the larger 10 French gauge probe at 30–40 W for 10 seconds.

These treatment devices share some common principles. All can be applied tangentially, but (apart from injection) are better used face-on if possible. When the vessel is actively bleeding, direct probe pressure on the vessel or feeding vessel will reduce the flow and increase the effectiveness of treatment (Fig. 5.18). The bipolar and heat probes incorporate a flushing water jet, which helps to prevent sticking.

• *Combination therapy* involves injection of epinephrine followed by application of thermal coaptive coagulation. This method appears superior to monotherapy for treatment of ulcers with active bleeding or adherent clots. Monotherapy remains sufficient for ulcers with a non-bleeding visible vessel.

• *Clipping* (Fig. 5.19). Metal clips can be applied endoscopically, and are particularly useful for small bleeding ulcers (e.g. Dieulafoy lesions), for Mallory–Weiss tears, and large visible vessels.

Know when to stop treatment!

Treatment attempts should not be protracted if major difficulties are encountered; the risks rise as time passes. There are some patients and lesions in which endoscopic intervention may be

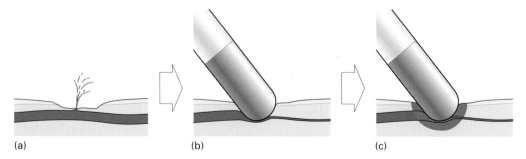

(a)   (b)   (c)

Fig 5.18 (a) Bleeding ulcer. (b) Probe pressure stops the blood flow and coapts the vessel wall. (c) Coagulation.

foolhardy, and surgery is more appropriate, for example, a large posterior wall duodenal ulcer that may involve the gastroduodenal artery. Angiographic treatment is useful in selected cases.

Follow-through after treatment

A single endoscopic treatment is not an all-or-nothing event. It is necessary to continue other medical measures, to maintain close monitoring, and to plan ahead for further intervention (pharmacological, endoscopic, radiological, or surgical) if bleeding continues or recurs. The job is not complete until the lesion is fully healed. IV, followed by oral, PPI post-endoscopic treatment and eradication of *Helicobacter pylori* should reduce the risk of late rebleeding.

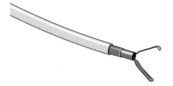

Fig 5.19 Hemostatic clip.

Treatment of bleeding vascular lesions

All of the endoscopic methods can be used to treat vascular malformations such as angiomas and telangiectasia. The risk of full-thickness damage and perforation is greater in organs with thinner walls (e.g. the esophagus and duodenum) than in the stomach. Lesions with a diameter of more than 1 cm should be approached with caution, and treated from the periphery inward to avoid provoking hemorrhage. Bipolar and heat probe and APC provide the best control.

Complications of hemostasis

The most important hazards of endoscopic hemostasis are pulmonary aspiration and provocation of further bleeding. It is difficult to know how often endoscopy causes rebleeding that would not have occurred spontaneously, but major immediate bleeding is unusual and can usually be stopped. The risk of pulmonary aspiration is minimized by protecting the airway using pharyngeal suction and a head-down position, or a cuffed endotracheal tube. Perforation can be caused by any of the treatment methods if they are used too aggressively, especially in acute ulcers, which have little protecting fibrosis.

Enteral nutrition

There are several ways in which endoscopists can assist patients who need nutritional help. Temporary support can be provided by placement of a nasoenteric feeding tube. Long-term nutritional support requires the creation of a gastrostomy (or jejunostomy).

Feeding and decompression tubes

Tubes for short-term feeding (and gastric decompression) are normally placed blindly at the bedside, but can also be passed under fluoroscopic guidance or after endoscopic placement of a guidewire. Two direct endoscopic methods can be used when necessary, for example to advance tubes through the pylorus or a surgical stoma. These are the ***through-the-channel method*** and the ***along-the-scope method***.

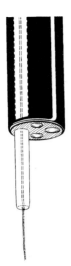

Fig 5.20 The feeding tube and guidewire are passed through a large-channel scope.

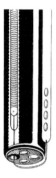

Fig 5.21 A tube is carried alongside the scope by a thread grasped with a snare or forceps.

Through-the-channel method

This is the simplest technique and entails advancing a 7–8 French gauge plastic tube through a large-channel endoscope, over a standard (400-cm-long) 0.035-inch diameter guidewire (Fig 5.20). The tube and guidewire are advanced through the pylorus under direct vision, and subsequent passage is checked by fluoroscopy. When the tip is in the correct position, the endoscope is withdrawn while further advancing the tube (and guidewire) through it. Finally, the guidewire is removed and the tube is rerouted through the nose. Another method is to pass a guidewire through the biopsy channel into position in the small bowel. The endoscope is then removed and a feeding tube is fed over the guidewire into position.

Alongside-the-scope method

This technique allows the placement of a tube larger than the endoscope channel. The feeding tube is stiffened with one or more guidewires. A short length of suture material is attached to the end of the tube and is grasped within the instrument channel with a snare (Fig 5.21). The endoscope is passed into the stomach and close to the pylorus. The snare and tube are then guided through the pylorus (or stoma) under direct vision. Once in position (checked by fluoroscopy), the thread is released and the endoscope is removed. The proximal end of the tube is rerouted from the mouth to the nose. The final position is checked by fluoroscopy, withdrawing any excess loops in the stomach.

A variant of this method has proven useful recently. The feeding tube (again stiffened with one or more guidewires) is passed through the nose and into the stomach. The endoscope is passed through the mouth, and is used to push the tip of the tube through the pylorus. The endoscope is then passed alongside the tube into the duodenum. The tube advances by the friction between the scope and the tube. The tube is held firmly at the nose, and the scope is withdrawn to the pylorus and then advanced again to push the tube deeper.

Percutaneous endoscopic gastrostomy (PEG)

Nasoenteric feeding can be used for several weeks but is inconvenient and unstable, and it is probably often responsible for pulmonary aspiration and pneumonia. PEG is now a popular method for long-term feeding, and may permit the transfer of patients with chronic neurological disability from acute care hospitals into nursing homes. The PEG technique can be extended into a feeding jejunostomy by the use of appropriate tubes.

Studies comparing PEG with operative gastrostomy have shown some advantages for the endoscopic method, but surgical (and laparoscopic) options should always be considered, especially in circumstances where the endoscopic approach may be more difficult or hazardous (e.g. after gastric surgery).

Antibiotics are usually given to reduce the risk of skin sepsis.

There are two main methods for PEG placement: the "pull" and the "push" methods.

The "pull" technique

This, the original method, is still the most commonly used.

1 *A standard endoscope is passed and the gastric outlet is checked.*

2 *The patient is rotated onto the back, the stomach distended with air, and the room darkened* (this is particularly important when using videoscopes).

3 *The tip of the endoscope is directed toward the anterior wall* of the stomach.

4 *The assistant observes the abdominal wall for transillumination* and indents the site with a finger.

5 *The endoscopist checks the indentation site* is in an appropriate part of the body of the stomach.

6 *The assistant marks this spot on the anterior abdominal wall*, applies disinfectant, and infiltrates local anesthetic into the skin, subcutaneous tissues, and fascia.

7 *A 5–10 mm skin incision is made* with a pointed blade, extending into the subcutaneous fat.

8 a: *The assistant inserts an 18 gauge needle catheter* (loaded onto a syringe half full of water) through the anterior abdominal wall, aspirating after initial penetration. Air should not bubble back until the needle is visible endoscopically (showing that it is in the stomach, not in another organ such as the colon).

8 b: *The endoscopist places a snare in front of the area of indentation and needle entry*, and maintains gastric distension.

8 c: *A string is passed through the needle and is grasped with the snare* (the string has loops at both ends and must be at least 150 cm long) (Fig 5.22a).

9 *The endoscope and snare are withdrawn through the mouth* (Fig 5.22b) carrying the string, while ensuring that the external end of the string remains outside the abdominal wall.

10 *The PEG tube is attached to the string loop coming out of the mouth, then pulled down the esophagus (Fig 5.22c) and through the anterior abdominal wall* (Fig 5.22d). The tube should not be pulled tight, to avoid compression necrosis of the gastric wall. Leave about 1 cm of "play," as judged endoscopically.

11 *The tube is shortened and then anchored at the skin* with one of various disk devices.

12 *Feeding can start on the day after the procedure* (with a trial of water initially) if there are no complications.

13 *The patient and all relevant caregivers are given detailed instructions* on tube care, and what to do if problems arise.

14 *After about 2 months the initial tube can usually be replaced* with a flat feeding button.

The "push" technique

This follows steps 1 through 8 above, to the point where the needle catheter is in the stomach, with the endoscope poised in front of it. A long straight guidewire is then pushed through the needle, and grasped endoscopically with a snare. The scope and snare are removed via the mouth, so that there is a long wire extending from the mouth through the stomach and through the abdominal wall. Keeping tension on both ends of the wire, a special PEG tube is

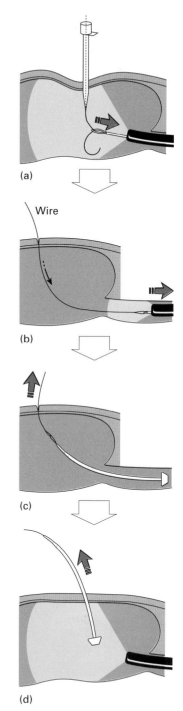

Fig 5.22 PEG. (a) Grasp the wire. (b) Pull the wire through the mouth. (c) Pull the PEG tube down the esophagus. (d) Pull bumper to gastric wall.

then slid all the way over the wire. The tip of the tube is grasped as it exits the abdominal wall, and pulled into place. An external bolster is attached.

Direct introducer technique

This is used in some countries, especially by radiologists. The feeding tube is pushed through the abdominal wall, rather than pulling it down from the mouth. The stomach is distended with air using a nasogastric tube under fluoroscopy. A needle catheter, trochar, and straight guidewire are passed through the abdominal wall into the stomach. A succession of dilators are passed over the wire, and eventually a PEG tube in a sleeve. The sleeve is removed and the PEG withdrawn into position. This method eliminates contamination of the PEG tube by passage through the mouth, but it is difficult to choose the correct puncture position unless endoscopy is used. It is sometimes also difficult to push the trochar and catheter through the abdominal and stomach walls. A new variant of this technique (PEX-ACT) uses specialized needles and loops to create sutures anchoring the stomach wall to the abdominal wall before insertion of the large-bore PEG tube. Again, this requires internal visualization using an endoscope.

PEG problems and risks

PEG placement cannot be performed in patients with esophageal strictures that are too tight to permit the passage of an endoscope. Technical difficulties and risks are higher in patients who have previously undergone abdominal surgery, particularly with partial gastric resection, and in patients with gastric varices, marked ascites, or obesity.

Specific risks of PEG

There are three main types of risk.
- *Perforation/fistula*. Avoid injuring other organs (such as the colon) by making sure that good transillumination is achieved, and by using the bubble-back check. A small pneumoperitoneum is not uncommon, and is usually benign, but major and persisting leakage requires operative correction.
- *Local infection* can occur (even necrotizing fasciitis), particularly if the skin incision is too small or if the tube has been pulled too tight against the gastric wall (one of the most common errors). Preprocedure antibiotics reduce this risk.
- *Tube dislodgement* can result in peritonitis and may require surgical repair. Dislodgement after 10–14 days usually leaves a track (for 12–24 hours) during which the tube can be replaced (with care).

Percutaneous endoscopic jejunostomy (PEJ)

Jejunal feeding is often recommended to reduce the risk of pulmonary aspiration, especially in patients with gastroesophageal reflux and gastroparesis. The jejunostomy tube may be inserted (under endoscopic guidance) through an established PEG tract or using special commercial kits at the time of the original PEG puncture (PEG-J). The technique for placing the tip of the tube in the jejunum is similar to the "alongside-the-scope" method for naso-jejunal tubes described above. Placing a jejunostomy tube directly into the small bowel, by analogous transillumination/puncture techniques, has been done and obviates the need for surgery or interventional radiology but does carry higher risks compared with PEJ/PEG-J.

Nutritional support

The purpose of these endoscopic interventions is to provide safe and effective nutritional support. It is thus important to ensure that the patient and all involved caregivers are instructed appropriately about tube care and feeding regimens. They also need structured follow-up support.

Further reading

Neoplasia

Allum WH, Blazeby JM, Griffin SM, Cunningham D, Jankowski J, Wong R. on behalf of the Association of Upper Gastrointestinal Surgeons of Great Britain and Ireland, The British Society of Gastroenterology, and the British Association of Surgical Oncology. Guidelines for the management of oesophageal and gastric cancer. *Gut* 2011; **60**: 1449–72.

American Society for Gastrointestinal Endoscopy. The Role of Endoscopy in the Assessment and Treatment of Esophageal Cancer. *Gastrointest Endosc* 2003; **57**: 817–22.

American Society for Gastrointestinal Endoscopy. Technology Status Evaluation Report. Enteral Stents. *Gastrointest Endosc* 2011; **74**: 455–64.

Leiper K, Morris AI. Treatment of oesophago-gastric tumors. *Endoscopy* 2002; **34**: 139–45.

Vermeijden JR, Bartelsman JFWM, Fockens P *et al*. Self-expanding metal stents for palliation of esophagocardial malignancies. *Gastrointest Endosc* 1995; **41**: 58–63.

Foreign bodies

American Society for Gastrointestinal Endoscopy. Guideline for management of ingested foreign bodies and food impaction. *Gastrointest Endosc* 2011; **73**: 1085–91

Quinn PG, Connors PJ. The role of upper gastrointestinal endoscopy in foreign body removal. In: *Gastrointestinal Endoscopy Clinics of North America* (series ed. Sivak MV). Philadelphia: WB Saunders, 1994, pp. 571–93.

Webb W. Management of foreign bodies of the upper gastrointestinal tract. *Gastroenterology* 1988; **94**: 204–16.

Nutrition

American Society for Gastrointestinal Endoscopy. Role of endoscopy in enteral feeding. *Gastrointest Endosc* 2011; **74**: 7–12.

DeLegge MH, Sabol DA. Provision for enteral and parenteral support. In: *Handbook of Clinical Nutrition and Aging* (eds Bales CW, Ritchie CS). Totowa, NJ: Humana Press, 2003, pp. 583–95.

Bleeding

American Society for Gastrointestinal Endoscopy. The role of endoscopic therapy in the management of variceal hemorrhage. *Gastrointest Endosc* 2005; **62**: 651–5.

American Society for Gastrointestinal Endoscopy. The role of endoscopy in the management of acute non-variceal upper GI bleeding. *Gastrointest Endosc* 2012; **75**: 1132–8.

Binmoeller KF, Soehendra N. "Super glue"; the answer to variceal bleeding and fundal varices? *Endoscopy* 1995; **27**: 392–6.

Cipolletta L, Bianco MA, Marmo R *et al.* Endoclips versus heater probe in preventing early recurrent bleeding from peptic ulcer: a prospective and randomized trial. *Gastrointest Endosc* 2001; **53**: 147–51.

Imperiale TE, Chalasani N. A meta-analysis of endoscopic variceal ligation for primary prophylaxis of esophageal variceal bleeding. *Hepatology* 2001; **33**: 802–7.

Iwase H, Maeda O, Shimada M *et al.* Endoscopic ablation with cyanoacrylate glue for isolated gastric variceal bleeding. *Gastrointest Endosc* 2001; **53**: 585–92.

Jalan R, Hayes PC. UK guidelines on the management of variceal haemorrhage in cirrhotic patients. *Gut* 2000; **46**(Suppl 3–4): 1–15.

Laine L, Peterson WL. Bleeding peptic ulcer. *N Engl J Med* 1994; **331**: 717–27.

Lau JY, Sung JJ, Lee KK *et al.* Effect of intravenous omeprazole on recurrent bleeding after endoscopic treatment of bleeding peptic ulcers. *N Engl J Med* 2000; **343**: 310–6.

Lau JY, Sung JJ, Lam YH *et al.* Endoscopic retreatment compared with surgery in patients with recurrent bleeding after initial endoscopic control of bleeding ulcers. *N Engl J Med* 1999; **340**: 751–6.

Lo GH, Lai KH, Cheng JS *et al.* Emergency banding ligation versus sclerotherapy for the control of active bleeding from esophageal varices. *Hepatology* 1997; **25**: 1101–4.

Messmann H, Schaller P, Andus T *et al.* Effect of programmed endoscopic follow-up examinations on the rebleeding rate of gastric or duodenal peptic ulcers treated by injection therapy: a prospective, randomized controlled trial. *Endoscopy* 1998; **30**: 583–9.

Rollhauser C, Fleischer DE. Nonvariceal upper gastrointestinal bleeding. *Endoscopy* 2002; **34**: 111–8.

Sarin SK, Mishra SR. Endoscopic therapy for gastric varices. *Clin Liver Dis* 2010; **14**: 263–79.

Scottish Intercollegiate Guidelines Network (SIGN). *Management of acute upper and lower gastrointestinal bleeding.* Guideline No 105. September 2008.

Esophageal

Ferraris R, Fracchia M, Foti M *et al.* Barrett's oesophagus: long-term follow-up after complete ablation with argon plasma coagulation and the factors that determine its recurrence. *Aliment Pharmacol Ther* 2007; **25**: 835–40.

Kostic S, Kjellin A, Ruth M *et al.* Pneumatic dilatation or laparoscopic cardiomyotomy in the management of newly diagnosed idiopathic achalasia: results of a randomized controlled trial. *World J Surg* 2007; **31**: 470–8.

Marchese M, Spada C, Costamagna G. Endoluminal fundoplication. *Minim Invasive Ther Allied Technol* 2006; **15**: 356–65.

Shaheen NJ. The rise and fall (and rise?) of endoscopic anti-reflux procedures. *Gastroenterology* 2006; **131**: 952–4.

General

Carr-Locke DA, Branch MS, Byrne WJ *et al.* Botulinum toxin therapy in gastrointestinal endoscopy. *Gastrointest Endosc* 1998; **47**: 569–72.

Carr-Locke DA, Conn MI, Faigel DO. Developments in laser technology. *Gastrointest Endosc* 1998; **48**: 711–6.

Cotton PB, Sung J. Advanced digestive endoscopy; upper endoscopy. www.gastroHep.com, posted 2003.

Giday SA, Kantsevoy SV, Kalloo AN. Principle and history of natural orifice translumenal endoscopic surgery (NOTES). *Minim Invasive Ther Allied Technol* 2006; **15**: 373–7.

Kantsevoy SV, Hu B, Jagannath SB *et al*. Technical feasibility of endoscopic gastric reduction: a pilot study in a porcine model. *Gastrointest Endosc* 2007; **65**: 510–3.

Kimmey MB, Al-Kawas F, Burnett DA *et al*. Electrocautery use in patients with implanted cardiac devices. *Gastrointest Endosc* 1994; **40**: 794–5.

Pasricha PJ, Fleischer DE, Kalloo AN. Endoscopic perforations of the upper digestive tract; a review of their pathogenesis, prevention and management. *Gastroenterology* 1994; **106**: 787–802.

Ponsky JL. Endoluminal surgery: past, present and future. *Surg Endosc* 2006; **20**(Suppl 2): S500–2.

Now check your understanding—go to

www.wiley.com/go/cottonwilliams/practicalgastroenterology

CHAPTER 6

Colonoscopy and Flexible Sigmoidoscopy

History

The history of colonoscopy (Video 6.1) started in 1958 in Japan with Matsunaga's intracolonic use of the gastrocamera under fluoroscopic control, and subsequently Niwa's development of the "sigmocamera." Not surprisingly, these instruments had application only in the hands of pioneer enthusiasts. Following Hirschowitz's development of the fiberoptic bundle in 1957–1960 for use in prototype side-viewing gastroscopes, several colorectal enthusiasts started developments. The first was Overholt in the USA, who started on prototypes in 1961, performed the first fiberoptic flexible sigmoidoscopy in 1963, and finally introduced a commercial forward-viewing short "fiberoptic coloscope" in 1966 (American Cystoscope Manufacturers Inc.). Meanwhile, Fox in the UK and Provenzale and Revignas in Italy had achieved imaging of the proximal colon with passive fiberoptic viewing bundles or side-viewing gastroscopes inserted through a tube placed radiologically or pulled up by a swallowed transintestinal "guide string and pulley" system.

In 1969 Western researchers were surprised by the production by Japanese engineers (Olympus Optical and Machida) of remarkably effective colonoscopes, which combined the precise two-way angulation and torque-stable shaft of the latest gastrocameras with superior fiberoptic bundles, although initially the limitations of Japanese glassfiber technology restricted angulation to around 90° (due to fragile fibers) and the angle of view to 70°.

Gastric snare polypectomy was first described by Niwa in Japan in 1968–9, and snaring of colon polyps was pioneered in 1971 by Deyhle in Europe and Shinya in the USA.

In the mid-1970s four-way acutely angulating instruments were introduced, and in 1983 the video endoscope arrived (Welch-Allyn, USA). Although small-scale colonoscope production continued for a time in the USA, Germany, Russia, and China, the combined mechanical, optical, and electronic know-how of the Japanese camera manufacturers now controls the conventional colonoscope market.

Indications and limitations

The place of colonoscopy in clinical practice depends on local circumstances and available endoscopic expertise. Although colonos-

Cotton and Williams' Practical Gastrointestinal Endoscopy: The Fundamentals, Seventh Edition.
Adam Haycock, Jonathan Cohen, Brian P Saunders, Peter B Cotton, and Christopher B Williams.
© 2014 John Wiley & Sons, Ltd. Published 2014 by John Wiley & Sons, Ltd.
Companion Website: www.wiley.com/go/cottonwilliams/practicalgastroenterology

copy is considered the "gold standard" exam, "virtual" colography by computed tomography (CT) or even double-contrast barium enema (DCBE) alone may be considered by some to be adequate in "low-yield" patients where therapeutic intervention, histology, or fine-focus diagnosis is not needed. Similarly, on the grounds of logistics, safety, and patient acceptability, flexible sigmoidoscopy has a significant role in clinically selected patients with minor symptoms and is being introduced as part of population colorectal cancer screening in the UK.

Double-contrast barium enema

DCBE is a safe (one perforation per 25 000 examinations) way of showing the configuration of the colon, the presence of diverticular disease, and the absence of strictures or large lesions. However, even high-quality DCBE has significant limitations, including missing large lesions because of overlapping loops (particularly in the sigmoid region), to misinterpreting between solid stool and neoplasm or between spasm and strictures, with particular inaccuracy for flat lesions such as angiodysplasia or minor inflammatory change and small (2–5 mm) polyps. Where colonoscopy services are overstretched, and CT colography is not routinely available, barium enema may be used in "low yield" patients—those with pain, altered bowel habit or constipation; it also shows extramural leaks or fistulae, which are invisible to the endoscopist.

Computed tomography colography

CT colography ("virtual colonoscopy") has replaced barium enema as the radiological investigation of choice for the colon, with the advantages of being quicker and not filling the colon with dense contrast medium. CT colography does require technical expertise of the radiographer in perfoming it and the radiologist who interprets it. A few patients who are very difficult to colonoscope for reasons of anatomy or postoperative adhesions may be best examined by combining limited left-sided colonoscopy—the most challenging area for imaging but with the highest yield of significant pathology—with virtual colography or barium enema to demonstrate the proximal colon. Virtual colography has the advantage that it can be performed before or after colonoscopy and with the same bowel preparation, although the majority of procedures are now performed with limited or no bowel preparation and "faecal tagging" using water-soluble contrast agents. CT colography requires radiation dosage comparable to that of DCBE, although dedicated CT protocols limit radiation as much as possible.

Colonoscopy and flexible sigmoidoscopy

Colonoscopy and flexible sigmoidoscopy achieve more than contrast radiology or virtual colography because of their greater accuracy and histologic and therapeutic capabilities. Color view and biopsy makes total colonoscopy particularly relevant to patients with bleeding, anemia, bowel frequency, or diarrhea. Flexible sigmoidoscopy alone may be sufficient for some patients, such as those with left iliac fossa pain or bright red per-rectal bleeding.

Table 6.1 Colonoscopy: indications and yield.

High-yield indications	Low-yield indications
Anemia/bleeding/occult blood loss	Constipation
Persistent diarrhea	Flatulence
Inflammatory disease assessment	Altered bowel habit
Genetic cancer risk	Pain
Abnormality on imaging	
Therapy	

Because of near pinpoint accuracy and therapy, colonoscopy scores for any patient at increased risk for cancer—in whom detection and removal of all adenomas is important for the patient's future and as a predictor of long-term risk. Colonoscopy is thus the method of choice for many clinical indications and for cancer surveillance examinations and follow-up (Table 6.1). Endoscopy is also particularly useful in the postoperative patient, either to inspect in close-up (and biopsy if necessary) any deformity at the anastomosis or to avoid the difficulties of achieving adequate distension in patients with a stoma.

Combined procedures

The combination of two procedures (colonoscopy and virtual colography or DCBE) has potential advantages. If carbon dioxide (CO_2) insufflation is used for colonoscopy or flexible sigmoidoscopy, the colon will be absolutely deflated within 10–15 minutes and DCBE can follow immediately. As distension is a routine part of virtual colography, it is an ideal procedure to combine with colonoscopy. DCBE can be made difficult if the proximal colon is already air-filled, so problematic to fill and coat with barium. Colonoscopic biopsies with standard-sized forceps are no contraindication to distending the colon for subsequent DCBE or CT colography. Pedunculated polypectomy should also be safe, but the likelihood of deep electrocoagulation during sessile polypectomy, however small, contraindicates use of distension pressure. DCBE perforation is rare, but barium peritonitis can be fatal.

Limitations of colonoscopy

• *Incomplete examination* can be due to inadequate bowel preparation, uncontrollable looping, inadequate hand-skills, or an obstructing lesion. Unless the ileo-cecal valve is reached and positively identified with clear views of the cecal pole, completion has not been proved.
• *Gross errors in colonoscopic localization and "blind spots" are possible* even for expert endoscopists. Blind areas, with the possibility of missing very large lesions, occur especially in the cecum, around acute bends and in the rectal ampulla. Colonoscopic examination, rigorously performed, can probably approach 90% accuracy for small lesions, but will never be 100%. A "back to back" colonoscopy series, in which the patient was colonoscoped twice

by two expert endoscopists, showed only a 15% miss rate for polyps under 1 cm diameter. However, every colonoscopist has experienced the chagrin of seeing a large polyp during insertion, but missing it entirely during withdrawal when the colon is crumpled after straightening the scope.

Hazards, complications, and unplanned events

Colonoscopy, despite its virtues, is more hazardous than diagnostic alternative studies (historically around one perforation per 1500 colonoscopic examinations, although much lower in recently published series, against perforations in 1:25000 barium enemas or CT colography exams). Unskilled endoscopists needing to use heavy sedation or general anesthesia to cover up ineptitude are likely to run greater risks. It should therefore not be regarded as failure to abandon a tough colonoscopy in favor of immediate CT colography, when "pressing on regardless" could result in an avoidable perforation and subsequent complications.

Instrument shaft or tip perforations

These perforations are usually caused by inexperienced users and the use of excessive force when pushing in or pulling out. In a pathologically fixed, severely ulcerated, or necrotic colon, however, forces that would be safe in a normal colon may be hazardous. Either the tip of the instrument or a loop formed by its shaft can perforate. Shaft loop perforations are characteristically larger than expected, so, if in doubt, surgery should be advised. When surgery has been performed soon after apparently uneventful colonoscopy, small tears have been seen in the ante-mesenteric serosal aspect of the colon and hematomas found in the mesentery. In other cases the spleen has been avulsed during straightening maneuvers when the tip is hooked around the splenic flexure.

Air pressure perforations

These include "blow-outs" of diverticula, "pneumoperitoneum," and ileo-cecal perforation following colonoscopy limited to the sigmoid colon. Surprisingly high air pressures result if the scope tip is impacted in a diverticulum or if insufflation is excessive, for instance when trying to distend and pass a stricture or segment of severe diverticular disease. Use of CO_2 insufflation minimizes these serious risks post-procedure, as it is so rapidly absorbed. Diverticula are thin-walled and have also been perforated with biopsy forceps or by the instrument tip. It is surprisingly easy to confuse a large diverticular orifice with the bowel lumen or to mistakenly identify an inverted diverticulum, usually in the proximal colon, as a small sessile polyp.

Hypotensive episodes

Hypotensive episodes, even cardiac or respiratory arrest, can be provoked by the combination of oversedation and the intense vagal stimulus of forceful or prolonged colonoscopy. Hypoxia is particularly likely in elderly patients, but should be a thing of the past if pulse oximetry (or CO_2 capnography) is routinely used and nasal oxygen given prophylactically to sedated patients.

Infection

As mentioned elsewhere, prophylactic antibiotics are rarely indicated before colonoscopy, then only for well-defined groups such as severely immunocompromised patients, and possibly those with ascites or on peritoneal dialysis. However, Gram-negative septicemia can result from instrumentation (especially in neonates or the elderly) and unexplained post-procedure pyrexia or collapse should be investigated with blood cultures and managed appropriately.

Management following complications

Therapeutic procedures inevitably increase the risk of complications, including dilatations (4% of which resulted in perforations in our series), electrocoagulation of bleeding points or sessile polypectomies. However, the hazards are remarkably infrequent compared with the morbidity and mortality considered acceptable for surgery. To generalize (and perhaps exaggerate), endoscopic misadventure risks surgery; surgical misadventure risks death. The endoscopist should therefore be on guard for problems that can occur and should only undertake therapeutic procedures with the knowledge of a back-up surgical team.

It is also worth remembering, however, that fatalities have also been reported after colonoscopic perforation followed by unnecessary surgery (rather than relying on conservative management with antibiotic cover). The decision whether or not to operate after a complication can be a subtle one, but the maxim should be "if in doubt, operate"—although the surgeon consulted needs to be aware of the particular endoscopic circumstances. Most therapeutic perforations will be small and occur in a well-prepared colon, so they may sometimes be considered for conservative management. For instance, perforation following point electrocoagulation of an angiodysplasia in the cecum has a reasonable chance of sealing off spontaneously (with the patient immobilized and on antibiotics). By contrast, an unexplained perforation after a difficult and forceful colonoscopy, especially if bowel preparation was poor, indicates exploratory surgery because there may be an extensive rent in the colon.

Safety

Safety during colonoscopy comes from gentle technique and avoiding pain (or oversedation, which masks the pain response as well as contributing pharmacological hazards). Before starting a colonoscopy it is impossible to know if there are adhesions, whether the bowel is easily distensible, and whether its mesenteries are free-floating or fixed; pain is the only warning that the bowel or its attachments are being unreasonably strained. The endoscopist must respect any protest from the patient; a mild groan in a sedated patient may be equivalent to a scream of pain without sedation. Moreover, it is hazardous to give repeated doses of sedatives intravenously, effectively anesthetizing the patient without an anesthetist being present. It is safer in such cases to abandon the procedure and reschedule as a formal anesthetic procedure. ***Total colonoscopy is not always technically possible, even for experts.***

If there is a history of abdominal surgery or sepsis, or if the instrument feels fixed and the patient is in pain, the correct course is usually to stop. The experienced endoscopist learns to take time, to be obsessional in steering correctly and managing loops dexterously, but to be prepared to withdraw from any difficult situation and if necessary to try again after position change or other appropriate maneuver. Too often the beginner has a relentless "crash and dash" approach, and may be insensitive to the patient's pain because it occurs so often.

Despite its potential hazards, skilled colonoscopy is amazingly safe; it is certainly justified by its clinical yield and the high morbidity of colonic surgery (which would often be the alternative). For the less skilled endoscopist, partnership with CT colography in "difficult" cases should reduce the risks—with re-referral to an expert if pathology is found.

Informed consent

Obtaining full informed patient consent is essential before an invasive procedure such as colonoscopy, with its potential for complications. The patient should understand the rationale for undergoing the procedure, its benefits, risks, limitations, and alternatives, and have an opportunity to ask the doctor any questions. Precise approaches to the explanation of risks vary from country to country, and should probably be tailored to some extent to the perceived insights and anxieties of the individual patient. Some patients wish to know everything, some would be distressed to have scary and unlikely minutiae (such as "the unlikely possibility of death") spelled out to them. Any possible complication with an incidence greater than 1:100 or 1:200 should certainly be explained, so that a frank discussion of the "pluses and minuses" of anticipated therapeutic procedures, such as removal of large sessile polyps or dilation of strictures, should be mandatory. Ideally, the endoscopist should quote personal figures and experience.

It is logical and our routine practice to mention to all adult patients the remote possibility of postpolypectomy delayed bleeding occurring for up to 14 days post-procedure, in case a polyp is found incidentally during colonoscopy and is judged to require removal (even though the procedure is scheduled as "diagnostic"). Most patients will acquiesce immediately, but a commonsense discussion of practicalities is relevant. A patient about to have a holiday in remote parts or organizing a family wedding or other major event may be disinclined to take any risk whatever—and would justifiably be aggrieved should a complication occur.

Contraindications and infective hazards

There are few patients in whom colonoscopy is contraindicated. Any patient who might otherwise be considered for diagnostic laparotomy because of colonic disease is fit for colonoscopy, and colonoscopy is often undertaken in very poor risk cases in the hope of avoiding surgery.

• *There is no contraindication to colonoscopy during pregnancy*, although it might be best avoided in those with a history of miscarriage.

• *There is no contraindication to the examination of infected patients* (e.g. patients with infectious diarrhea or hepatitis) because all normal organisms and viruses should be inactivated by routine cleaning and disinfection procedures. Mycobacterial spores require a longer disinfection, so, after the examination of suspected tuberculosis patients and before/after the examination of AIDS patients (possible carriers of mycobacteria) prolonged disinfection is recommended (see Chapter 2).

• *Antibiotic prophylaxis is unnecessary*, according to current UK and US guidelines, even after heart valve replacement or previous bacterial endocarditis. It may be indicated in severely immunocompromised patients (see Chapter 2).

• *Colonoscopy is absolutely contraindicated* during, and for 2–3 weeks after, *acute diverticulitis*, due to the risk of perforation from the localized abscess or cavity. It should not be performed, or only with the greatest care and minimal insufflation, in any patient with marked *abdominal tenderness, peritonism, or peritonitis*.

• *Colonoscopy is relatively contraindicated* for 3 months after *myocardial infarction*, when it is unwise owing to the risk of dysrhythmias.

• *Colonoscopy is relatively contraindicated in patients with known ascites or on peritoneal dialysis* because of the probability of scope pressure causing transient release of bowel organisms into the bloodstream and peritoneal cavity.

• *Colonoscopy should only be undertaken with good reason and extreme care when there is acute or severe inflammation* (ulcerative, Crohn's or ischemic colitis), especially if abdominal tenderness suggests an increased risk of perforation. If large and deep ulcers are seen it may be wise to limit or abandon the examination. After irradiation, especially a year or more after exposure, narrowed or obstructed bowel can be perforated without using excessive force. If insertion proves difficult it may be best to withdraw or to change to a smaller instrument.

• *Other factors can be relevant* and should be considered during the process of obtaining information and consent, including previous medical history and current medications. For obvious reasons, medications such as anticoagulants or insulin may affect management. A cardiac pacemaker theoretically contraindicates use of magnetic imaging or argon plasma coagulation (APC) but these should not affect modern insulated pacemakers. Patients with implantable defibrillators, however, are at risk from inappropriate firing of their devices during standard diathermy. These patients require full cardiac monitoring during electrosurgery, with a technician available to switch their device before and after the procedure.

Patient preparation

Most patients can manage bowel preparation at home, arrive for colonoscopy, and walk out shortly afterwards. Management routines depend on national, organizational, and individual factors. Overall management is influenced, among other things, by:
- cost
- facilities available
- type of bowel preparation and sedation used
- age and state of the individual patient
- potential for major therapeutic procedures
- availability of adequate facilities and nursing staff for day-care and recovery.

Experienced colonoscopists in private practice or large units are motivated to organize streamlined day-case routines, even for patients with large polyps. Some nationalities (Dutch, Japanese) do not expect sedation, whereas others (British, American) frequently insist on it. In countries with sufficient anesthesiologists (France, Australia) use of propofol or full general anesthesia has, regrettably in our opinion, become the norm for colonoscopy. These variables result in an extraordinary spectrum of performance around the world, from the many skilled colonoscopists who require patients for less than an hour on a "walk-in, walk-out" basis in an office or day-care unit, to others with less experience and a traditional hospital background who feel that many hours in hospital, or even an overnight stay, are essential.

Colonoscopy can be made quick and easy for the majority of patients. This requires both a reasonably planned day-care facility and an endoscopist with the confidence and skill to work gently and reasonably fast. Some flexibility of approach is wise. A very few patients are better admitted before or after the procedure. The very old, sick, or very constipated may need professional supervision during bowel preparation. Frail patients may merit overnight observation afterwards if their domestic circumstances are not supportive or they live far away. We do rarely admit a few patients for polypectomy, especially if the lesion is very large and sessile and the patient has a bleeding diathesis or is unavoidably on anticoagulants or antiplatelet medications (clopidogrel, etc.). Even such patients, however, providing they live near good medical support services and have been fully informed about what to do in a crisis, can often be justifiably managed on an outpatient basis, as complications are rare and can in any case be "delayed" several days post-procedure.

Bowel preparation

An informed team member should be available to talk to the patient at the time of booking to explain the procedure, including the importance of successful bowel preparation—although printed instructions and explanations will be sufficient for most patients. The majority of patients find that the worst part of colonoscopy is the bowel preparation and that the anticipation of the procedure (including fear of indignity, a painful experience, or the possible findings) is much worse than the reality of the colonoscopy itself. Anything that will justifiably cheer them up beforehand is extremely worthwhile, providing that there is understanding and compliance with dietary modification and bowel preparation. Minutes spent in explanation and motivation may prevent a prolonged, unpleasant, and inaccurate examination due to bad preparation. The patient needs to know that a properly prepared colon looks as clean and easy to examine as the mouth—whereas poor preparation can lead to a degradingly unpleasant, less accurate, and slower examination.

Written dietary instructions are well worthwhile, as many patients, anxious to get a good result, find it easier to follow specific instructions "to the letter." Clear instructions avoid unnecessary anxieties and many telephone calls.

Limited preparation

Enemas alone are usually effective for limited colonoscopy or flexible sigmoidoscopy in the "normal" colon. The patient need not diet and typically has one or two disposable phosphate enemas (e.g. Fleet Phospho-soda®, Fletchers', Microlax), self-administered or given by nursing staff. Examination can be performed shortly after evacuation occurs—usually within 10–15 minutes—so that there is no time for more proximal bowel contents to descend. The colon can often be perfectly prepared to the transverse colon in younger subjects (NB in babies phosphate enemas are contraindicated because of the risk of hyperphosphatemia). Note that patients with any tendency to faint or with functional bowel symptoms (pain, flatulence, etc.) are more likely to have severe vaso-vagal problems after stimulant enemas; make sure they are supervised or have a call button. Lavatory doors should be able to be opened from and toward the outside in case the patient should faint against the door.

Diverticular disease or stricturing requires full bowel preparation even for a limited examination, because bowel preparation will be less effective and enemas less likely to work.

If obstruction is a possibility, per oral preparation is dangerous, even potentially fatal. In ileus or "pseudo-obstruction" normal preparation simply does not work. One or more large-volume enemas are administered in such circumstances (up to 1 L or more can be held by most colons). A contact laxative such as oxyphenisatin (300 mg) or a dose of bisacodyl can be added to the enema to improve evacuation (see below).

Full preparation

The object of full preparation is to cleanse the whole colon, especially the proximal parts, which are characteristically coated with surface residue after limited regimens. However, patients and colons vary. No single preparation regime predictably suits every patient, and it is often necessary to be prepared to adapt to individual needs. Constipated patients need extra preparation; those with severe colitis may be unfit to have anything other than a warm saline or tap water enema. A preparation that has previously proved unpalatable, made the patient vomit, or that failed is unlikely to be a success on another occasion—a different one should be substituted. Recommendations are now published by respective societies on suitability for bowel preparation. Current data support "split-dose" administration (see below) to increase acceptability and resultant success of preparation.

Dietary restriction is a crucial part of preparation. The patient should have no indigestible or high-residue food for 24–48 hours before colonoscopy (avoiding muesli, fibrous vegetables, mushrooms, fruit, nuts, raisins, etc.). Staying on clear fluids for 24 hours is even better if the patient is compliant, but is not really necessary. Soft foods that are easily digested (soups, omelettes, potato, cheese, and ice-cream) can be eaten up to (and including) lunch on the day preceding colonoscopy. Only supper and breakfast before colonoscopy need to be replaced with fluids. Tea or coffee (with some milk if wanted) can be drunk up to the last minute, since minor fluid residues present no problem to the endoscopist.

Drink extra clear fluids—the more the better! Fruit juices or beer are found by many to be easier to drink in large quantities than water, and white wine or spirits can also help morale during the fasting phase. However, *red wine is discouraged* because it contains iron and tannates and, when digested with other dietary tannates, causes the bowel contents to become black, sticky, and offensive. Any other clear drink, water ices or sorbets (not blackcurrant), consommé (hot or cold), boiled sweets, or peppermints can all be taken up to the last minute. There is no reason why anyone should feel ravenous or unduly deprived of calories by the time of colonoscopy.

Medications or supplements containing iron should be stopped at least 3–4 days before colonoscopy, as organic iron tannates produce an inky black and viscous stool, which interferes with inspection and is difficult to clear. *Constipating agents* should also be stopped 1–2 days before.

Most medications can be continued as usual, except for modification of anticoagulant regimens and withdrawal of clopidogrel and similar platelet-inhibiting agents for one week before planned polypectomy.

PEG-electrolyte preparation

Balanced electrolyte solution with polyethylene glycol solution (PEG) is very widely used. This is primarily because it has formal approval from the US Food and Drug Administration (FDA) (e.g. GoLYTELY®, NuLYTELY®, CoLyte®, KleenPrep®, etc.) and comes with suitable flavorings, convenient packaging, and is easily prescribed, but it is surprisingly expensive. Although the PEG component of a PEG–electrolyte mixture contributes the majority of the packaged weight, volume, and expense, it results in only a minority of the osmolality (sodium salts being, of physiological necessity, the important component). Even chilled, its taste is mildly unpleasant due to the Na_2SO_4, bicarbonate, and KCl included to minimize body fluxes. Modification of the original formula by omitting Na_2SO_4 and reducing KCl only slightly improves the taste. A further recent variant, apparently popular and effective, is MoviPrep®, which combines PEG–electrolyte with ascorbic acid (aspartame, the sweetening agent used in it, can be nauseating to some patients).

Patient acceptance of PEG–electrolyte oral preparation can be enhanced, without impairing results from the endoscopist's point of view, by the simple expedient of administering the volume necessary in two half doses ("split administration"), with most drunk the evening before but the rest on the morning of the examination (see "Routine" below). There are conflicting reports about whether the addition of prokinetic agents or aperients improves results; the consensus is that it does not.

Mannitol

Mannitol (and similarly sorbitol or lactulose) is a disaccharide sugar for which the body has no absorptive enzymes. It is available ready-made as intravenous (IV) solutions that can be drunk. Mannitol solution is an isosmotic fluid at 5% (2–3 L) or acts as a hypertonic purge at 10% (1 L) with a corresponding loss of electrolyte and body fluid during the resulting diarrhea, although this is only of concern in the elderly and normally can be rapidly reversed by drinking. The solution's sweetness can be nauseous to those without a sweet tooth, although this is much reduced by chilling and adding lemon juice or other flavorings. Children, in particular, tend to vomit it back. Mannitol solution alone (1 L of 10% mannitol drunk iced over 30 minutes, followed by 1 L of tap water) is a useful way of achieving rapid bowel preparation (in 2–3 hours) for those requiring urgent colonoscopy.

There is a potential **explosion hazard** after mannitol, because colonic bacteria possess the necessary enzymes to metabolize carbohydrates to form explosive concentrations of hydrogen. Electrosurgery should therefore be covered by CO_2 insufflation or all colonic gas conscientiously exchanged several times by aspiration and re-insufflation.

Magnesium salts

Magnesium citrate and other magnesium salts are very poorly absorbed, acting as an "osmotic purge." The gently cathartic properties of "spa" waters rich in magnesium salts, such as Vichy water, have been known since Roman times. Picolax®, a proprietary combination, produces both magnesium citrate (from magnesium oxide and citric acid) and bisacodyl (from bacterial action on sodium picosulfate). It tastes acceptable and works well in most patients. Taking 2–3 bisacodyl tablets in addition improves results, but can cause cramping.

For seriously constipated patients, magnesium sulfate, although unpleasant-tasting, is highly effective if taken in repeated doses (5 mL of crystals in 200 mL hot water every hour, followed by juice and other fluids). It can be guaranteed eventually "to move mountains."

Sodium phosphate

Sodium phosphate, presented as a flavored half-strength equivalent of the phosphate enema (Fleet's Phospho-Soda®) but administered orally, has received numerous good reports when trialed against 4 L PEG–electrolyte preparation. It is said to be as effective as PEG–electrolyte solution but is significantly more acceptable to patients, principally because the volume ingested is only 90 mL. Although the taste is generally disliked, this has been partially solved by the introduction of Phospho-Soda tablets. Sodium phosphate must be followed by at least 1 L of other clear fluids of choice—water, juices, lager, etc. Because concerns remain about the risk of significant electrolyte disturbances (hypokalemia, hypocalcemia, hyperphosphatemia), which could initiate cardiac arrythmias, sodium phosphate is unsuitable for those with any degree of renal impairment, which includes most elderly patients.

Routine for taking oral prep

Low-residue diet instructions should have been followed, ideally for several days in the case of those with known constipation or slow transit. The patient should be supplied with petroleum jelly or barrier cream to avoid perianal soreness (colorless to avoid endoscope lens contamination as the scope is inserted through the anus). The evening before colonoscopy will be fluid-dominated—input and output—so social events should not be scheduled but there will be plenty of time for watching television or reading between "calls."

As mentioned above, large-volume solutions are ideally split-administered in two doses, starting on the afternoon or evening before, but *it is essential that some oral prep is taken on the morning of the examination* so that cecal contents remain fluid and easily aspirated. If an afternoon examination is scheduled and the patient does not have a long distance to travel, both doses can be drunk on the day of examination.

The patient should be encouraged to carry on with normal activities, rather than sitting still during the drinking period; exercise stimulates transit and evacuation. Bowel actions should start within 1–3·hours, but can be much delayed in constipated patients or those who prove to have a long colon.

Bowel preparation in special circumstances

Children

Children usually accept pleasant-tasting oral preparations such as senna syrup or magnesium citrate very well. Drinking large volumes is less well accepted, and mannitol may cause nausea or vomiting. The childhood colon normally evacuates easily except, paradoxically, for colitis patients, who prove perversely difficult to prepare properly. Small babies may be almost completely prepared with oral fluids plus a saline enema. Phosphate enemas are contraindicated in babies because of the possibility of hyperphosphatemia.

Colitis patients

Colitis patients require special care, during and after preparation. Relapses of inflammatory bowel disease occasionally occur after overvigorous bowel preparation but balanced PEG–electrolyte solutions are well tolerated. A simple tap water or saline enema will clear the distal colon sufficiently for limited colonoscopy. Patients with severe colitis are unlikely to need colonoscopy at all, as plain abdominal x-ray, ultrasonography, or scanning will usually give enough information.

For severely ill patients any distension is risky and colonoscopy is positively contraindicated due to the potential for perforation. When the indication for colonoscopy in a colitis patient is to exclude cancer or to reach the terminal ileum to help in differential diagnosis, full and vigorous preparation is necessary.

Constipated patients

Patients with constipation often need extra bowel preparation. This is very difficult to achieve in patients with true megacolon or Hirschsprung's disease, in whom colonoscopy should be avoided if at all possible. Constipated patients should have 48 hours on low-residue diet, as they normally take a high-fiber regime but have slow transit. They should continue any habitually taken purgatives in addition to the regime for colonoscopy preparation.

Colostomy patients

Colostomy patients are as difficult to prepare as normal subjects. Oral preparation is well tolerated, whereas enemas/colostomy washouts are tedious and difficult for nursing staff to perform satisfactorily, unless the patient is accustomed to this and can do it for themselves.

Stomas, pouches, and ileo-rectal anastomoses present few problems. Ileostomies are self-emptying and normally need no preparation other than perhaps a few hours of fasting and clear fluid intake. Ileo-anal pelvic pouches can be managed either by saline enema or by reduced volume of oral lavage. After ileo-rectal anastomosis, the small intestine can adapt and enlarge to an amazing degree within some months of surgery, so that if the object of the examination is to examine the small intestine, full oral preparation should be given. For a limited look, any conventional enema is usually enough (NB stimulant enemas sometimes cause vaso-vagal response).

Defunctioned bowel, for instance the distal loop of a "double-barreled" colostomy, always contains a considerable amount of viscid mucus and inspissated cell debris, which will block the colonoscope. Conventional tap water or saline rectal enemas or tube lavage through the colostomy are needed to clear a defunctioned bowel. Hypertonic (phosphate) or stimulant enemas will be less effective.

Colonic bleeding

Active colonic bleeding helps preparation, as blood is a good purgative. Some patients requiring emergency colonoscopy may need no specific preparation at all, providing that examination is started during the phase of active bright red bleeding. Position change during insertion of the instrument will shift the blood and create an air interface through which the instrument can be passed. Changing to the right lateral position clears the proximal sigmoid and descending colon, which is otherwise a blood-filled sump. Actively bleeding patients requiring preparation for more accurate total colonoscopy can be managed by nasogastric tube lavage, which allows examination within an hour or two and ensures that blood is washed out distal to the bleeding point, rather than carried proximally with enemas. Blood can be refluxed to the terminal ileum from a left colon source, which makes localization difficult unless it is being constantly washed downward by a per-oral high-volume preparation. Massively bleeding patients can be examined per-operatively with on-table colon lavage combining a cecostomy tube with a large-bore rectal suction tube (and bucket), but more often should be managed angiographically with no preparation at all.

Medication

Attitudes to medication differ greatly from country to country. We favour adapting to the individual patient.

Sedation and analgesia

All aspects of the procedure, including the medication options, should be explained when the colonoscopy booking is arranged. The patient should receive preliminary verbal and written explanation about bowel preparation and what to expect of the procedure (whether from doctor, nurse, or secretary). At this point some patients may judge (in countries where judgment is permitted) that they want full medication, others that they will hope to work normally or to drive afterwards. On arrival for colonoscopy, a few minutes of further explanation will reassure and calm most patients and allow the endoscopist to judge whether the particular individual is likely to require sedation, and if so how much. Most people tolerate some discomfort without resentment if they understand the reason for it. Few people expect to be semi-anesthetized for a visit to the dentist, but on the other hand they understandably expect the intensity and duration of any discomfort to be within "acceptable limits." Pain thresholds and individual attitudes to pain are not always easy to predict before colonoscopy, because tolerance of the (peculiarly unpleasant) quality of visceral pain varies so much. It is sensible to warn the patient that there will be a few seconds of "wind" or a transient sensation of "urgency."

During a typical and correctly performed colonoscopy, minor pain is experienced by the patient for only 20–30 seconds. Using moderate or no sedation, and employing the skills, changes of position, and other "tricks of the trade" described below, pain only occurs during looping in the sigmoid colon and while passing the sigmoid–descending colon junction. During the rest of a normal procedure a patient with average pain threshold should experience little more than mild distension or the urge to pass flatus. It is worth pointing out to the patient that pain is useful to the endoscopist because it shows that a loop is forming, but is not dangerous and can usually be stopped in a few seconds (by straightening out the loop that is causing it).

The use of sedation has advantages and disadvantages. The unsedated or very lightly sedated patient can cooperate by changing position, needs no recovery period, and can travel home unaided immediately. The colonoscopist is also encouraged to develop dexterous and gentle insertion technique. On the other hand, some endoscopists who never employ sedation also admit to only 80–90% success in performing total colonoscopy, presumably because some examinations are intolerable. If light "conscious sedation" is used (typically equivalent in effect to 2–3 glasses of wine or beer), the patient is likely to find the examination tolerable or to have amnesia for it. The endoscopist is helped to be thorough by the knowledge that the patient is comfortable, and is also more likely to achieve total colonoscopy in a shorter time. Using heavy sedation, endoscopists can get away with ham-handed and forcibly looping technique—a bad investment in the long term, less likely to achieve complete examinations, more likely to result in complications, and more expensive in instrument repair bills.

It is often said that it is dangerous to sedate, because the safety factor of pain is removed. This is not strictly true, providing that the endoscopist's threshold of awareness lowers as the patient's pain threshold is raised—taking restlessness or changes of facial expression as a warning that tissues and attachments are being overstretched.

Most endoscopists use a balanced approach to sedation that will be affected by many factors, including personal experience and the individual patient's attitude. A relaxed patient with a short colon having a limited examination rarely needs sedation, but an anxious patient with a tortuous colon, severe diverticular disease, or a bad previous experience, may need deep sedation. Patients with irritable bowel syndrome or pain as presenting features are likely to be hypersensitive to stretch and will benefit from opiates.

A very few patients have a morbid fear of colonoscopy, a low pain threshold, or a known "difficult" colon that justifies offering light general anesthesia. General anesthesia is only likely to be hazardous if it allows an inexperienced colonoscopist to use brutal technique while the patient cannot protest. However, even experienced endoscopists are more likely to "push the limits" and to become more mechanistic if patients are routinely anesthetized and "out of it."

Nitrous oxide inhalation

Nitrous oxide/oxygen inhalation can be a useful "half-way house" between no sedation and conventional IV sedation, for instance in a patient intending to drive after the procedure. The 50:50 nitrous oxide/oxygen mixture is self-administered by the patient, inhaling from a small cylinder fitted with a demand valve. Breathing the gas through a small single-use mouthpiece (Fig 6.1) avoids the difficulties that can be experienced in getting a good fit with a face mask, and also the phobia that some patients experience with masks.

The patient is shown how to inhale, then "pre-breathes" for a minute or two as the endoscopist prepares to start the procedure, with the intention of achieving gas saturation of the body fatty tissues. Thereafter it takes only 20–30 seconds of gas breathing, when required, to obtain a "high" that makes short-lived pain

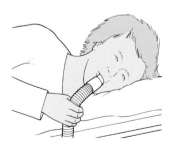

Fig 6.1 Nitrous oxide/oxygen mixture is breathed through a mouthpiece.

significantly more tolerable. Nitrous oxide/oxygen inhalation should prove useful for some flexible sigmoidoscopies and, used alone, can be sufficient for motivated patients having total colonoscopy by a skilled endoscopist. Scared patients, prolonged or difficult examinations and examinations by inexpert endoscopists require conventional sedation.

Intravenous sedation

The ideal sedative regime for colonoscopy would last only 5–10 minutes, with a strong analgesic action but no respiratory depression or after-effects, allowing the patient to be comfortable yet accessible and able to change position during the procedure, but then to recover rapidly afterwards. The nearest approach to this ideal is currently given by IV delivery, through an in-dwelling plastic cannula, of a benzodiazepine hypnotic such as midazolam (Versed® 1.25–5 mg maximum) or diazepam (Valium® 2.5–10 mg maximum) either given alone or combined with a low dose of an opiate such as pethidine (meperidine 25–100 mg maximum) or fentanyl (50–100 mg). The benzodiazepine produces anxiolytic, sedational, and amnesic effects while the opiate contributes analgesia and (especially relevant to pethidine) a useful sense of euphoria.

In general, only a small dose of benzodiazepine should be given unless the patient is very anxious. The initial injection is given slowly over a period of at least 1 minute, "titrating" the dose to some extent by observing the patient's conscious state and ability to talk coherently—some patients merely become loquacious. A small initial "starter dose" makes it possible to judge during initial insertion through the sigmoid whether the rest of the procedure is likely to be easy or difficult, and whether the patient is pain-sensitive or not. Half dosage in total is used for older, sicker patients but the amount required is unpredictable; younger patients may tolerate maximal doses and remain (fairly) coherent. If in doubt it is safer to underestimate the titration and give more later if necessary.

Use extra opiate rather than more benzodiazepine if extra medication is needed. Benzodiazepines make some patients even more restless and have no painkilling properties. Benzodiazepines and opiates potentiate each other, not only in effectiveness but also in side effects such as depression of respiration and blood pressure. Pulse oximetry should therefore be routinely used, and in most units nasal oxygen is administered in all sedated patients—with the caveat that this is contraindicated in severe chronic obstructive airways disease, where CO_2 capnography would ideally be used.

• *Benzodiazepines* have a useful mild smooth-muscle antispasmodic action as well as their anxiolytic effect. Diazepam (Valium®) is poorly soluble in water and the injectable form is therefore carried in a glycol solution that can be painful and cause thrombophlebitis, especially if administered into small veins. For this reason, it is better to use water-soluble midazolam (Versed®). Midazolam causes a greater degree of amnesia, which can be useful to cover a traumatic experience but also "wipes" any explanation of the findings, which must be repeated later on. It should be borne in mind that IV midazolam dosage should be half that of diazepam.

- *Opiates* (pethidine notably) induce a useful sense of euphoria in addition to their analgesic efficacy. Pethidine may cause local pain when administered through small veins, particularly in children, but this can largely be avoided by diluting the injection 1:10 in water. A mild, symptomless small-vein phlebitis may be seen in a small minority of patients but invariably resolves spontaneously with no need for treatment. Pentazocine (Fortral®) is a weaker analgesic, more hallucinogenic and seems to have little to recommend it. Fentanyl (Sublimaze®) is very short-lived, so is strongly favoured by some endoscopists although it gives no sense of well-being, unlike pethidine.
- *Propofol* (Diprivan®), a short-lived IV emulsion anesthetic agent, is widely used for colonoscopy in some countries (USA, France, Germany, Australia) and increasingly in others. It should ideally be administered by an anesthetist because of the significant risk of marked respiratory depression but, with appropriate training and safeguards, has been extensively employed by endoscopists with an anesthetic-trained nurse assistant, with apparent safety and satisfactory results. Its short duration of action—giving full recovery within about 30 minutes—is an advantage over excessive doses of conventional sedatives. However, the patient can be rendered insensible and unable to cooperate with changes of position or to give early warning of excessive pain. We therefore prefer to reserve the use of propofol for selected patients having particular requirement for transient "heavy sedation"—usually because of previous difficulty or pain-sensitivity, or because of an anticipated problematic procedure.

Antagonists

The availability of antagonists to benzodiazepines (flumazenil) and opiates (naloxone) is invaluable, providing a safety measure for occasions when inadvertent oversedation has occurred. Some endoscopists routinely administer antagonists (intravenously and/or intramuscularly) to reduce the recovery period, which suggests mainly that their "routine" dosage regime is excessive. We use flumazenil extremely infrequently, but periodically administer naloxone intramuscularly on reaching the cecum if the patient appears oversedated. The patient is then conveniently awake by the time the examination is finished, without the risk of later "rebound" re-sedation, which is reported after IV naloxone wears off.

Antispasmodics

Antispasmodics induce colonic relaxation for at least 5–10 minutes and help to optimize the view during examination of a hypercontractile colon. Either hyoscine *N*-butylbromide (Buscopan®) 20 mg IV (in countries where it can be prescribed) or glucagon 0.5–1 mg IV are effective. Fears about anticholinergics initiating glaucoma are misplaced because patients previously diagnosed are completely protected by their eye drops, and those with undiagnosed chronic glaucoma are best served by precipitating an acute attack, which will cause the diagnosis to be made. Patients should be told to seek medical attention if they experience any eye pain. Glucagon is more expensive, but has no ocular or prostatic side effects.

Intravenous antispasmodics have a relatively short duration of action, leading some endoscopists to give them only when the colonoscope is fully inserted. Experienced endoscopists, sure of a rapid procedure, may give them at the start. There is an unproven suspicion that the bowel is rendered more redundant and atonic by antispasmodics and will be more difficult to examine; on the contrary, we find that the view is improved and have shown that colonoscope insertion is speeded up after using antispasmodics. Benzodiazepines have a weak antispasmodic effect, relaxing most colons except for those that are "irritable" or spastic. In the unsedated patient, therefore, antispasmodics may be particularly helpful and can also be a useful placebo for those who cannot have routine sedation because they need to drive home, but expect an "injection" to cover the procedure.

Insufflation with CO_2 avoids post-procedure problems, especially in patients with irritable bowel disorder or diverticular disease. If air is used such patients can experience problems from air retention, with sudden onset of colic or discomfort after the procedure as the pharmacological effects of the antispasmodics and sedation wear off.

Equipment—present and future

This chapter aims to "make colonoscopy easy," but this also depends to a fair degree on the instrumentation used. We have tried to generalize and be noncommercial in approach, as the colonoscopes of all manufacturers are serviceable and we have used many of them—although with individual preferences. A number of ingenious innovations are under current evaluation, designed to propel or guide the colonoscope or to view the colon more easily. While enthusiastic for future improvements and innovations, we have deliberately excluded these from the present account, which describes the best ways to manage the "push" colonoscopes currently used, including those with in-built stiffening or "magnetic imaging" facilities.

Colonoscopy room
Most units perform colonoscopies in undesignated endoscopy rooms, because the only special requisite for colonoscopy is good ventilation to overcome the evidence of occasional poor bowel preparation. In a few patients with particularly difficult and looping colons it has in the past been helpful to have access to x-ray facilities, especially in teaching institutions. Magnetic imaging (see below) performs the same function without using x-rays; it is increasingly used. We hope that it will spread worldwide to help teaching and the logical performance of colonoscopy.

Colonoscopes
Colonoscopes are engineered similarly to upper gastrointestinal endoscopes, but are longer, have a wider diameter (for better twist or torque control), and have a more flexible shaft. The bending

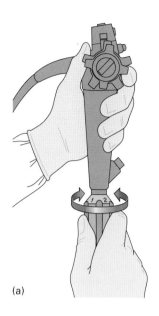

(a)

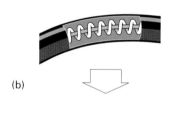

(b)

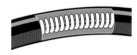

(c)

Fig 6.2 (a) Variable-stiffness colonoscopes have a twist control on the shaft. A pull-wire within an internal spring-steel coil (b) compresses the coil and stiffens it (and the scope) (c).

section of the colonoscope tip is longer and more gently curved, avoiding impaction in acute bends such as the splenic flexure. Ideal future colonoscopes ought to have electronic steering to make single-handed insertion easier; present angulation control mechanisms are almost unchanged from those of early gastrocameras and gastroscopes and are poorly suited to the more finicky steering movements during colonoscopy.

The introduction of variable stiffness instruments avoids the need to choose the "right colonoscope for the job" at the stage of purchase or before starting examination of a particular patient—especially one known or predicted to have a long "difficult" colon or severe adhesions. Long colonoscopes (165–180 cm) are able to reach the cecum even in redundant colons and so are our preferred routine choice of instrument (see also "variable-stiffness colonoscopes" below). Intermediate-length instruments (130–140 cm) are considered by some, including most German or Japanese endoscopists, to be a good compromise, almost always reaching the cecum. The only advantage of using 70-cm flexible sigmoidoscopes for limited examinations is that the endoscopist knows from the onset that the procedure will be limited, so avoiding the temptation to go further. However, as flexible sigmoidoscopy can be performed with a longer instrument (a pediatric colonoscope is ideal) there is no reason to purchase flexible sigmoidoscopes for an endoscopy unit, although they may have an essential role in the office of a primary-care physician or an outpatient facility.

Variable-stiffness colonoscopes

Variable-stiffness colonoscopes (Innoflex®, Olympus Corporation) have a twist control on the shaft (Fig 6.2a) that forcibly compresses and rigidifies an internal steel coil similar to that in a bicycle brake cable (Fig 6.2b,c Video 6.2). Compressing the coil stiffens it and the shaft/insertion tube within which it lies. The last 30 cm to the tip of the bending section is left "floppy" at all times. The bonus of using a variable-stiffness colonoscope is that, without having to withdraw and exchange instruments, the endoscopist can select a relatively "floppy" shaft mode to pass looping sections of the colon, then twist to apply "stiff" mode, so discouraging re-looping after the scope has been straightened out, typically at the splenic flexure.

Variable-stiffness scopes thus combine, in one colonoscope, many of the virtues of both standard and pediatric instruments. They prove significantly easier and less traumatic to use in most patients found previously to be "difficult" to examine—especially where the problem was due to uncontrollable looping and discomfort. As any first-time patient may prove to be difficult, a long, variable-stiffness instrument is our "colonoscope of choice."

Pediatric colonoscopes

Pediatric colonoscopes of small diameter (9–10 mm) are available with either standard, "floppy," or variable-shaft characteristics. They are invaluable for the examination of babies and children up to 2–3 years of age but also have a role to play in adult endoscopy and are the preferred choice of some skilled endoscopists. As well as allowing examination of strictures, anastomoses, or stomas that would be impassable with the full-sized colonoscope, they are often much easier to pass through areas of tethered postoperative adhesions or severe diverticular disease. The pediatric colonoscope bending section is more flexible, making it easier to obtain a retroverted view of some awkwardly placed polyps, whether in the distal or proximal colon, in order to ensure complete removal. Floppy pediatric instruments are also particularly comfortable and easy to insert to the splenic flexure, tending to conform to the colon in a spontaneous spiral configuration, which avoids difficulty in passing to the descending colon.

For limited adult examinations, as for strictures or diverticular disease, a pediatric gastroscope can also be used (it has the bonus of an even shorter bending section, but the disadvantage of limited downward angling capability). The stiff shaft of a gastroscope, however, makes it less suitable than the pediatric colonoscope for examinations of small children and babies.

Instrument checks and troubleshooting

The functionality of the colonoscope should be checked before examination, because imperfections can be difficult to spot or tedious to remedy during it. Colonoscopy can be difficult enough without adding problems in instrument performance.

Insufflation/lens washing checks are essential before every colonoscopy. Because air flow and water wash share a short common exit channel (see Fig 2.5) the quickest way of simultaneously checking air/water functionality is to depress the water-wash valve and look for a healthy squirt from the scope tip. Once the procedure has started it is difficult to assess inadequacy of air flow and insufflation pressure, the resulting poor view making it seem that the colonoscopy is "difficult" or the colon apparently "hyper-contractile." A great deal of wasted time can be avoided by noticing any such problem before starting, and correcting it or changing instruments.

If there is no insufflation at all, check the light source. Is the air pump switched on? Are the umbilical and water-bottle connections pushed in fully and the water bottle screwed on? Is the rubber O-ring in place on the water-bottle connection? Is the air/water valve in good condition and seated properly (or the CO_2 valve in position where relevant), as it will otherwise allow air leakage? If in doubt, proper air insufflation pressure and flow can be proven by blowing up a rubber glove wound over the scope tip.

Water-wash failure is unusual, except because of an empty water bottle or a faulty air/water valve.

Suction failure can be caused by valve blockage, which should be obvious on careful inspection or changing the valve, or by debris blocking the suction channel. If this is in the shaft it can be dislodged by water-syringing through the biopsy port. Removing the suction valve and covering the opening on the control head with a finger is a quick way of improving suction pressure and can result in rapid clearance of the whole system (as when sucking polyp specimens). Applying the sucker tube directly to the suction-channel opening can also be effective in clearing particulate debris. As a final resort the whole suction system can be cleared by retrograde-syringing using a 50-mL bladder syringe and tubing attached to the suction port on the umbilical. Push the suction valve and also cover the biopsy port during this procedure to avoid unpleasant (refluxed) surprises.

Accessories

All the usual accessories are used down the colonoscope, including biopsy forceps, snares, retrieval forceps or baskets, injection needles, cytology brushes, washing catheters, dilating balloons, etc. Long and intermediate-length accessories work equally well down shorter instruments, so it is sensible to order all accessories to suit the longest instrument in routine use. Other manufacturers' accessories also work down any particular instrument and, as some are better than others, it is worth taking advice from colleagues when buying replacements.

Carbon dioxide

Few colonoscopists, regrettably, use CO_2 insufflation, although its use has much to commend it. CO_2 was originally used instead of air because of the explosive potential of colonic gases during electrosurgery. However, with the exception of bowel preparation using mannitol, the prepared colon has been shown to have no residual explosive gas. Nonetheless, even for routine examinations, the use of CO_2 offers the striking advantage that it is cleared from the colon 100 times faster than air (through the circulation, to the lungs and then breathed out). This means that 10–15 minutes after finishing an exam using CO_2 insufflation, the colon and small intestine are free of any gas and the patient's abdomen is deflated, whereas air distension can remain and cause abdominal bloating and discomfort for many hours, which is especially distressing for irritable bowel patients. In the unlikely event of perforation or gas leak (pneumoperitoneum), air under pressure would add to the hazard, whereas rapidly absorbed CO_2 and a well-prepared colon should markedly reduce it.

Any patient with ileus, pseudo-obstruction, stricturing, severe colitis, diverticular disease, or functional bowel disorder should benefit from the added safety and comfort of using CO_2 rather than air insufflation.

Low-pressure, controlled-flow CO_2 delivery systems with fail-safe pressure-reducing features are available commercially. These remove any risk of the patient being exposed to the hazard of high pressure from the cylinder in the event of failure of the conventional flow-meter. A CO_2 insufflation valve can be substituted for the usual air/water valve, but in practice it is easier to connect the CO_2 supply to the water bottle (Fig 6.3) and use the normal air/water valve, as the modest leakage of CO_2 into room atmosphere is of no more consequence than having another person in the room.

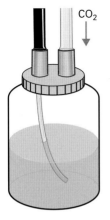

CO_2

Fig 6.3 Connect the CO_2 supply directly to the water bottle.

Magnetic imaging of endoscope loops

There is a need to know what shaft loops have formed during colonoscope insertion and where the tip is. In 1993 two UK groups introduced prototype magnetic imagers to "position-sense" the configuration of the instrument shaft, producing a moving 3D image on a computer monitor. Small coils within the instrument (or in a probe passed down its instrumentation channel) generate pulsed magnetic fields that energize larger sensor coils in a dish alongside the patient, computed to produce a real-time monitor graphic display (Fig 6.4). Two systems are commercially available: ScopeGuide® (Olympus Corporation) (Video 6.3), which uses coils incorporated within the shaft of the scope, and a catheter-based system inserted down the accessory channel of an ordinary colonoscope (Fujinon Magnetic Endoscopic Imaging). These produce fields no stronger than those of a television set and are safe for continuous use, except for patients with cardiac pacemakers.

In use, magnetic imaging makes many previously difficult and looping colons much quicker and easier to intubate, and also ensures that the endoscopist knows at all times where the colonoscope tip has reached and what loops have formed. It rationalizes many of the uncertainties of colonoscopy, and can be a boon to both beginners and experts. The magnetic imager is particularly helpful in patients with a long colon, who can be preselected on the basis of a history of constipation or the presence of hemorrhoids, or if they report a delayed response to bowel preparation.

Other techniques

Several other simple and straightforward amendments to standard insertion techniques are beginning to find favour. Water-immersion colonoscopy entails filling the colon with water to "smooth out" the floppy haustra and create a relatively straight colon. Cap-assisted colonoscopy uses a clear plastic cap attached to the tip of the colonoscope to assist with negotiating tight bends and can improve mucosal visualization on withdrawal. There are also many novel technologies in development to improve insertion and inspection (such as computer-controlled bending scopes, called retroscopes), but are not yet in routine use and are therefore currently beyond the remit of this book.

Anatomy

Embryological anatomy (and "difficult colonoscopy")

The embryology of colon development is complex and somewhat unpredictable, especially in terms of its outcome for mesenteries and fixations, which probably explains the extraordinarily variable configurations into which the colon can be pushed during colonoscopy (Video 6.4). The fetal intestine and colon initially develop as a functionless muscle tube joined at its midpoint to the yolk-stalk. This muscle tube lengthens into a U-shape on a longitudinal

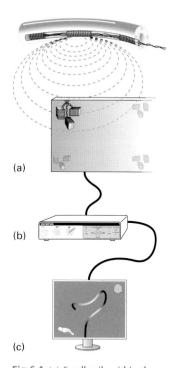

(a)

(b)

(c)

Fig 6.4 (a) Small coils within the scope generate magnetic fields, (b) energizing larger coils in the receiver dish beside the patient; (c) the signals are then processed as a 3D image on the monitor.

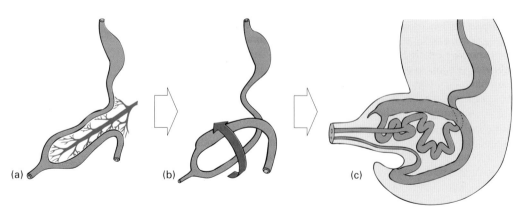

Fig 6.5 (a) The fetal intestine and colon start on a longitudinal mesentery (b) then rotate as the small intestine elongates (c) and from 5 weeks (1 cm embryo) to 10 weeks (4 cm embryo) are in the umbilical hernia.

mesentery (Fig 6.5a). As the embryo at this 5-week stage is only 1 cm long, the lengthening intestine and colon (Fig 6.5b) are forced out into the umbilical hernia (Fig 6.5c). The gut loop thus differentiates into the small and large intestine outside the abdominal cavity. By the third month of development the embryo is 4 cm long and there is room within the peritoneal cavity for first the small, and then the large, intestine to be returned into the abdomen. This occurs in a fairly predictable manner, with the end result that the colon is rotated around so that the cecum lies in the right hypochondrium and the descending colon to the left of the abdomen (Fig 6.6a).

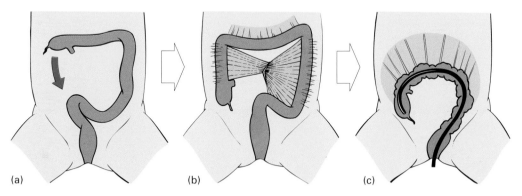

Fig 6.6 (a) The embryonic colon extends on its mesentery, (b) then partial fusion of the mesentery and peritoneum occurs at 3 months, (c) although sometimes the colon remains mobile.

With further elongation of the colon, the cecum normally migrates down to the right iliac fossa. At this stage, the mesentery of the transverse colon is free but the mesenteries of the descending and ascending colon, pushed against the peritoneum of the posterior abdominal wall by the fluid-filled and bulky small intestine, fuse with it so that the ascending and descending colon typically becomes retroperitoneal and fixed (although not always—see below) (Fig 6.6b).

Incomplete fusion of the mesocolon to the posterior wall of the abdomen results in a relatively free-floating colon. Such a mobile colon can be a nightmare for the colonoscopist, because there are no fixed points at which to obtain leverage, and few of the usual "tricks of the trade" will work, as most of them depend on withdrawal and leverage against fixations. The explanation for this variation from normal development may be the failure of enteric innervation of the intestinal muscle tube in early embryonic development. An atonic, bulky, and dysfunctional fetal intestine and colon will be retained longer than usual outside the abdomen in the umbilical hernia, until the developing abdominal cavity is large enough to re-accommodate it. Delayed return of a large colon into the abdomen will cause it to miss the "milestone moment" for retroperitoneal fixation and fusion to occur (usually by 10–12 weeks after conception). The long, mobile (and increasingly dysfunctional) colon may present clinically in childhood with straining at stool and bleeding, in teenage years with constipation, or in adulthood with hemorrhoids, variable bowel habit, and flatulence.

Endoscopically such a colon is noted to be unusually capacious, long, and often atypically looping, but it can also be dramatically squashed down and shortened when the colonoscope is withdrawn at the cecum (typically to a length of only 50–60 cm), proving the lack of fixations. Suggestive evidence that this is a genetically determined abnormality of development is the frequency of other first-degree relatives (especially on the female side and sometimes over several generations) known to have disturbance of habit, constipation, or flatulence. If endoscoped or imaged, the colon of such relatives (also their stomach and small intestine) are found to be similarly large, long, and mobile.

How often such failure of fusion, persistent colonic mesentery and mobility occurs is not clear from the literature. A persistent descending mesocolon has been found at postmortem in 36% with an ascending mesocolon in 10%. The persistence of a descending mesocolon explains most of the excessive loops and strange configurations that can be caused by the colonoscope passing the left colon and splenic flexure (Fig 6.7). Occasionally the cecum fails to descend and becomes fixed in the right hypochondrium (Fig 6.8); in others, where a free mesocolon persists, the cecum is mobile and can be pushed into weird configurations by the endoscope (Fig 6.9). Per-operative studies that we have undertaken show that colons in Asian patients are more predictably fixed than those in European patients.

Endoscopic anatomy

The *anal canal*, 3 cm long, extends up to the squamocolumnar junction or "dentate line." Sensory innervation, and hence mucosal pain sensation, may in some subjects extend up to 5–7 cm into the distal rectum. Around the canal are the anal sphincters, normally in tonic contraction. The anus may be deformed, scarred, or made sensitive by present or previous local pathology, including

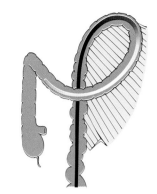

Fig 6.7 Persistent descending mesocolon or mesentery.

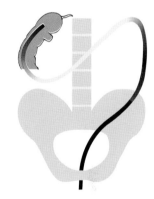

Fig 6.8 Inverted cecum.

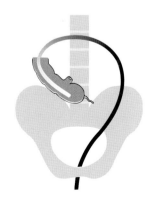

Fig 6.9 Mobile cecum.

hemorrhoids or other conditions. Normal subjects may also be sore from the effects of bowel preparation.

There are two potentially serious consequences from the fact that the hemorrhoidal veins drain into the systemic (not the portal) circulation:

1 Mistakenly snaring a "pile" can result in catastrophic hemorrhage.

2 Injecting intramucosal epinephrine (adrenaline) at a concentration greater than 1 : 200 000 before sessile polypectomy in the distal rectum has a serious risk of inducing potentially fatal cardiac or circulatory events (whereas the colonic vasculature drains via the portal system, so the liver metabolizes the higher concentrations of epinephrine often used proximally).

The **rectum**, reaching 15 cm proximal to the anal verge, may have a capacious "ampulla" in its mid-part as well as three or more prominent partial or "semilunar" folds (valves of Houston) that create potential blind spots, in any of which (as well as the distal rectum) the endoscopist can miss significant pathology. Digital examination, direct inspection and, where appropriate, a rigid rectoscope/proctoscope are needed for complete examination of the area. "Video-proctoscopy" (anoscopy—see below) is a convenient way of visualizing the anal canal, rectal mucosal prolapse, or hemorrhoids, but not the remainder of the rectum (which requires inflation for careful inspection and, where possible, instrument retroversion). Prominent, somewhat tortuous, veins are a normal feature of the rectal mucosa and should not be confused with the rare, markedly serpiginous veins of a hemangioma or the distended, tortuous varices seen in some cases of portal hypertension.

The rectum is extraperitoneal for its distal 10–12 cm, making this part relatively safe for therapeutic maneuvers such as Endoscopic Submucosal Dissection removal (see below) of sessile polyps. Proximal to this it enters the abdominal cavity, invested in peritoneum. Whereas the colon surface is devoid of sensory nerves and pain-free, patients may experience "burning pain" for up to 5–7 cm above the anal verge. This is easily managed for polypectomy by intramucosal local anesthetic injection.

Mucosal "microanatomy" is visible to the discerning endoscopist. This includes the shiny surface coating of mucus, around 30% of the mucosal cells being mucus-secreting and described as "goblet cells" because of their flask-shaped mucus-containing inclusions. The "highlights" reflected off the surface by the protective mucus layer can show up fine underlying detail, such as the arc impressions of circular muscle fibers or the dappled, sieve-like reflections caused by the microscopic crypt or pit openings. Minor abnormalities, such as prominent lymphoid follicles and the smallest polyps or flat adenomas, often first catch the endoscopist's eye through such reflections or "light reflexes" off the mucus layer. The mucosal columnar epithelium, around 50 cells thick, is transparent (unlike the horny squamous epithelium of the skin surface) and through it can be seen, often in exquisite detail, the paired venules and arterioles that make up the normal submucosal "vessel pattern."

Colonic musculature develops into three external longitudinal muscle bundles, or teniae coli, and within these, the wrapping of circular muscle fibers. Both muscle layers are sometimes visible to the endoscopist (Fig 6.10). One or more of the teniae may be seen endoscopically as a longitudinal fold, because an unusually thin-walled, capacious colon can bulge out between its teniae. The circular musculature is seen as fine reflective corrugations under the mucosal surface, particularly in "spastic" or hypertonic colons. The distal colon, needing to cope with formed stools, has markedly thicker circular musculature than in the proximal colon, resulting in a tubular appearance (Fig 6.11) broken by the ridged indentations of the haustral folds. The thinner walled transverse colon is kept in triangular shape by the three teniae.

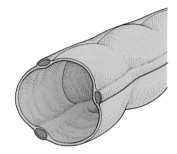

Fig 6.10 The longitudinal muscle bundles (teniae coli) can bulge visibly into the colon.

Haustral folds segment the interior of the colon. Those that are prominent in the proximal colon sometimes create "blind spots," whereas they can be hypertrophied in sigmoid diverticular disease, also creating mechanical difficulties for the endoscopist.

In elderly subjects the sigmoid colon anatomy is often narrowed and deformed internally by the thickened circular muscle rings of hypertrophic diverticular disease, and sometimes also fixed externally by pericolic post-inflammatory processes or adhesions. Redundant and prolapsing mucosal folds overlying the muscular rings in diverticular disease may appear reddened from traumatization, and sometimes show focal inflammation histologically as well.

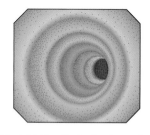

Fig 6.11 The distal colon is usually circular, with ridged haustrations.

External structures can be seen through the colonic wall, typically as the blue-gray discoloration of the spleen or the liver proximally. Vascular pulsations of the adjacent left iliac artery are often visible in the sigmoid, and right iliac artery pulsations are occasionally visible proximally. Marked aortic or cardiac pulsation can be seen in the transverse colon. Small intestinal gas distension or peristaltic activity may occasionally be visible through the colon wall, especially when it indents the cecal pole.

Insertion

Pre-procedure checks should be made on all functions of the endoscope, light source, and accessories before insertion (see above). A clean lens and correct color (white balance of the charge-coupled device (CCD)) are also important.

Insertion through the anus should be gentle. The instrument tip is unavoidably blunt (the lenses mean that it cannot be streamlined) so too fast or forcible insertion may be painful for patients with tight sphincters or a sore anal region. The squamous epithelium of the anus and the sensory mechanisms of the anal sphincters are the most pain-sensitive areas in the colorectum.

 There are several ways of inserting the scope (Video 6.5).

• *Start with two gloves* on the right hand and perform a digital examination with a generous amount of lubricant before inserting the instrument, both to check for pathology in this potentially "blind" area and to prelubricate and relax the anal canal. The

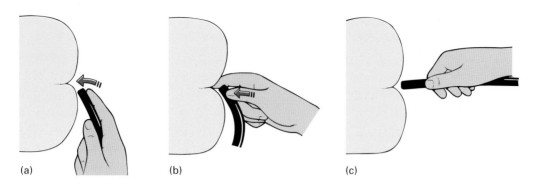

(a)   (b)   (c)

Fig 6.12 Different methods of colonoscope insertion: (a) finger support of the bending section; (b) the tip pushed in as the examining finger withdraws; or (c) straight on through the jelly.

instrument tip is passed in pressed in obliquely, supported by the examiner's forefinger until the sphincter relaxes (Fig 6.12a).

• *Use the thumb to push the tip in* along the examining forefinger as this withdraws from the anal canal (Fig 6.12b). The tendency of the bending section to flex can be avoided by starting with it straight, fixing the angulation control brakes and pressing in gently.

• *In the "direct" approach*, a large blob of lubricant jelly is spread over the anal orifice and the instrument is inserted directly through it (Fig 6.12c), which saves a glove and a few seconds. Inflating air down the endoscope while pressing the tip into the anal canal gives direct vision and facilitates insertion.

Tight or tonic sphincters may take time to relax; asking the patient to "bear down" is said to help this. Allowing an extra 15–20 seconds for sphincter relaxation can be a humane start to proceedings, especially for a patient with anorectal pathology or anismus. The sphincters of colitis patients are noticeably more tonic than normal, presumably because of the long-standing need to keep control and avoid leakage.

Video-proctoscopy/anoscopy

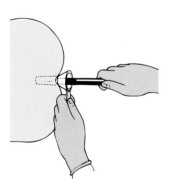

Fig 6.13 Video-proctoscopy (anoscopy).

Rigid proctoscopy has an important role in selected patients with bleeding after "normal colonoscopy" to inspect the anorectal area for mucosal prolapse, hemorrhoids, or other pathology. The patient can also be shown the anal canal or hemorrhoidal appearances by the simple expedient of inserting the video endoscope tip up the proctoscope once its insertion trocar is removed (the rectum will deflate and is poorly seen). The colonoscope simultaneously provides a convenient source of illumination and an excellent way of showing the patient any skin tags, anal papillae, or other local features that they could not normally see. The endoscopist performs this *video-proctoscopy or anoscopy* (Fig 6.13) from the monitor view, with the opportunity for taking a videotaped or printed record. In many cases of "unexplained bleeding" this will convincingly show the patient the likely (hemorrhoidal or mucosal) traumatic source of the problem.

Rectal insertion

A "red out" is often the first view after the scope has been inserted into the rectum. This is because the lens is pressed against the rectal mucosa. The following steps should be performed, in sequence (Video 6.5).

1 *Insufflate air* to distend the rectum.

2 *Pull back and angulate* or rotate slightly to find the lumen. This is the first of many times during the examination when withdrawal, inspection, and cerebration bring success more quickly than pushing blindly.

3 *Rotate the view* so that any fluid lies inferiorly. The suction port of the colonoscope tip lies just below the bottom right-hand corner of the image (Fig 6.14) and should be selectively placed in the fluid before activating the suction valve. Coordination will be required between shaft rotation (with the right hand) and synchronous up or down angulation (with the left hand) so as to keep the view. During examination *a skilled single-handed endoscopist often uses twist to torque-steer or "corkscrew" the tip*. The capacious rectum is the ideal place in which to practice this, as the shaft is inevitably straight and no force should be needed for precise finger-control.

4 *Aspirate fluid or residue* to avoid any chance of anorectal leakage during the rest of the examination. The warm, lubricated colonoscope shaft moving in and out often gives the patient a distressing illusion of being incontinent. Knowing that there is no rectal fluid to leak out and that any gas can be passed without fear of an accident is a bonus for everyone (not least the endoscopist).

5 *Push in*, finally, but only when an adequate view has been obtained, and only as fast as a reasonable view can be obtained.

6 *Torque-steer round* the first few bends, using up or down angulation and shaft-twist alone to achieve most lateral movements, rather than unnecessarily using the lateral angulation control. "Torque-steering" (with controlled shaft-twisting or corkscrewing movements) is an essential part of skilled colonoscopy.

Retroversion

Retroversion can be important in the rectum because, being relatively capacious, it can be surprisingly difficult to examine completely, even with a wide-angle lens. Care is needed to combine angulating and twisting movements sufficiently to see behind the major folds, or valves of Houston. In a capacious rectum the most distal part is a potential blind spot, but the generous size of such a large rectal ampulla will usually make tip retroflexion relatively easy. To perform it:

1 *pull back to the widest part of the distal rectum*

2 *angulate both controls fully*

3 *twist the shaft vigorously and simultaneously*

4 *push inward to invert the tip toward the anal verge* (Fig 6.15).

Retroversion is not always possible in a small or narrowed rectum, but when this is the case the wide-angled (130°, nearly "fish-eye") lens of the endoscope should see everything with minimal risk of blind spots.

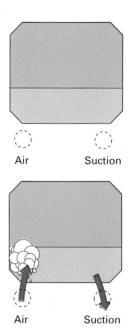

Air   Suction

Air   Suction

Fig 6.14 The colonoscope suction/instrumentation port opens below and to the right of the view; the air port below and to the left.

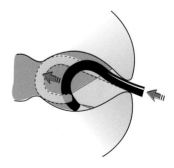

Fig 6.15 Angulate both controls, twist and *push in* to retrovert in the rectum.

Handling—"single-handed," "two-handed," or two-person?

Most skilled endoscopists favor the one-person "single-handed" approach, in which the colonoscopist manages the angulation controls and valves with one hand and inserts or twists the shaft with the other (Video 6.5). However there are many who use two hands on the angulation controls and a few experts who work successfully with the "two-person" method, using an assistant to manipulate the shaft.

Two-person colonoscopy

Two-person colonoscopy relies on an assistant to handle the shaft while the endoscopist uses both hands to manage the control body of the instrument, with the left hand working the up/down angulation control and air/water/suction valves but the right hand adjusting the right/left angulation control. Colonoscope control ergonomics are based on those of gastroscopes (and originally gastrocameras) and so are fundamentally designed for "two-handed" steering. However, whereas the short and stiff insertion tube of a gastroscope is easy for the endoscopist to control, the long and floppy shaft of a colonoscope is not. In this approach the assistant therefore performs the role delegated to the right hand of the single-handed endoscopist, pushing and pulling according to the spoken instructions of the endoscopist. A good assistant learns to feel the shaft to some extent and may apply some twist. More often, however, the assistant pushes with concealed gusto and causes unnecessary loops that are not apparent to the endoscopist, but painful for the patient.

Unless endoscopist/assistant teamwork is skilled and interactive, the two-person approach to colonoscopy can be as illogical and clumsy as would be expected of two people attempting any other intricate task, neither quite knowing what the other is doing.

In occasional difficult situations, for instance when passing an awkward angulation or snaring a difficult polyp, any endoscopist may justifiably involve the assistant briefly to steady or control the shaft. Otherwise, for the generality of colonoscopy, we do not recommend the two-person handling approach.

"Two-handed" one-person technique

The "two-handed technique" is a common compromise approach, the endoscopist using both hands on the angulation controls when required, but also handling the shaft for insertion and torque control. The two-handed approach is mainly used by those with small hands, who find it difficult to activate the lateral angulation control except by use of the right hand. Each time a lateral angulation is made the endoscopist has briefly to let go of the instrument shaft, which results in some loss of shaft control and "feel," with a tendency to jerky insertion. Some endoscopists ingeniously compensate by fixing the colonoscope shaft between thigh and couch whenever the right hand is steering.

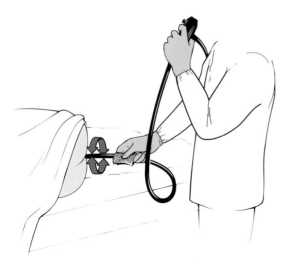

Fig 6.16 Single-handed maneuvering of the instrument shaft.

Occasional use of two-handed steering is entirely appropriate, but if the right hand is used too often for lateral angulations the endoscopist cannot torque-steer efficiently. Equally, if the right hand is away from the shaft for too long the endoscopist is being indecisive—it takes at most a second or two to make an angulation control adjustment and return the hand to shaft management.

"Single-handed" one-person colonoscopy—torque-steering

In "single-handed" colonoscopy, which we favor, the endoscopist manages all aspects of the colonoscope control body (angulation controls, valves, and switches) primarily with the left hand, leaving the right hand free to hold the shaft (Fig 6.16). This gives the endoscopist superior control and the opportunity to feel the colonoscope interacting with loops and bends.

• *Stance should be relaxed, holding the colonoscope in a relaxed manner*. Colonoscopy mostly requires fine and fluent movements, like those of a violin player, so a similarly balanced position and handling are needed.

• *Grip the shaft (insertion tube) 25–30 cm away from the anus*. Many endoscopists make the mistake of holding too close to the anus, resulting in the need for frequent changes of hand-grip and jerky insertion technique. Holding the shaft further back makes for smoother insertion, easier application of torque (maintained twisting force) and better feel of the forces involved.

• *Hold the shaft in the fingers*, with a gauze for cleanliness and extra friction, to feel and manipulate the shaft deftly. Finger-grip (Fig 6.17, Video 6.5) is used for delicate movements and exact control (as for a key or a small screwdriver), as opposed to the clumsier fist-grip used for a hammer or large screwdriver. Finger-grip makes it easier to feel whether the shaft is moving easily (is

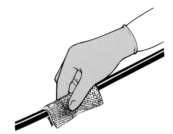

Fig 6.17 The instrument shaft should mostly be held delicately, in a gauze for added friction and feel, between the thumb and fingers.

Middle 'helper' finger

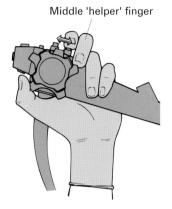

Fig 6.18 Single-handed control: the forefinger alone activates the air/water and suction valves; the middle finger is kept as "helper" to the thumb for major angulations.

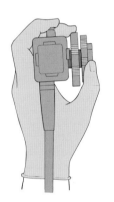

Fig 6.19 The thumb can reach the lateral angulation control (if the hand is positioned appropriately).

straight) or there is resistance (a bend or loop). Rolling the shaft between fingers and thumb allows shaft rotations of up to 360°, compared with a maximum of 180° achievable by wrist-twist.

• *Use a gauze or hand towel* to give better shaft feel and friction, whilst avoiding slippage from lubricant and improving cleanliness.

• *Discipline the fingers of the left hand* (Fig 6.18). Gripping the control body with only two fingers—the fourth (ring finger) and the little finger—lets the middle finger assume an invaluable role as "helper" to the thumb. Most endoscopists, unthinkingly but unnecessarily, use three fingers to hold the control body, and therefore find full angulation movements awkward. Single-handed steering is also made easier if the first finger alone operates the air/water or suction valves, which also leaves the middle finger free help the thumb manage the angulation controls. For those with reasonably large hands it is practicable for the left thumb to reach both the up/down or the lateral angulation controls (Fig 6.19).

• *Coordinate left- and right-hand activities*. The endoscopist is like a puppeteer propelling a snake puppet by the tail, with control of its head and a view through its eyes, but scant idea of what is happening to the snake's body—because this is invisible within the abdomen. For single-handed endoscopy, in order to control the snake fluently and efficiently, each hand must be disciplined to fulfill its appropriate tasks. The left hand supports the control body, manages the air/water/suction valves and the up/down angulation control (Fig 6.16), and adds minor thumb adjustments of left/right angulation when needed (Fig 6.19). The right hand should provide the artistry of skilled colonoscopy, with sensory feedback as well as deft movements. Because the colon is a continuous series of short bends and convolutions, requiring multiple combinations of tip angulation and shaft movement and frequent air/water and suction valve activations, any small delays and uncoordinated movements rapidly summate, prolonging the procedure unnecessarily.

• *Steer carefully and cautiously*. Steering movements should be early, slow, and exact (rather than jerky and erratic). A slow start to each angulation movement allows it to be terminated within a few degrees if the result is tip movement in the wrong direction. A rapid steering movement in the wrong direction can lose the view altogether, and then tends to be ineffectually corrected by another large movement. Flailing around is unnecessary and inelegant. Each individual movement should be slow and intentional.

• *Torque steering* involves first angulating up or down as appropriate and then, rather than using the lateral angulation control, torquing (twisting, rotating) the instrument shaft clockwise or counterclockwise with the right hand. Because the tip is angulated this rotation should corkscrew it around laterally (Fig 6.20, Video 6.5), precisely and quickly, and will often make use of the lateral angulation control unnecessary. Torque steering is, inevitably, affected by the direction in which the tip is angulated. "Up-angulation" with clockwise torque moves the tip to the right, whereas it moves to the left if angulation is down. Torquing is also a valuable way of orienting the scope tip in order to suction fluid efficiently or target lesions accurately (see Fig 6.14), so making biopsy-taking or polypectomy quicker and easier.

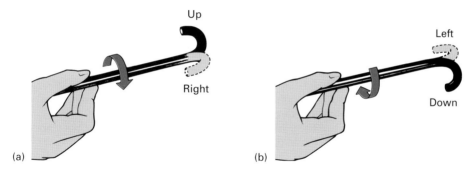

Fig 6.20 With a clockwise shaft twist: (a) an up-angulated tip moves toward the right, (b) whereas a down-angulated tip moves to the left.

- *Torque steering only works when the shaft is straight* (Fig 6.21a). When a loop is present in the shaft, twisting forces applied to it will be lost within the loop (Fig 6.21b). With the shaft straight, twist becomes an excellent way to torque or corkscrew around bends. Twist is particularly useful if a bend is acute or fixed, when trying to push around will be likely to result in shaft looping rather than tip progress.
- *Torque control of a loop prevents torque steering*. The principles of loop control are discussed below, when application of shaft torque force helps to straighten a spiral loop. Releasing "loop torque" (clockwise or counterclockwise) in order to "torque steer" in the other direction will allow the loop to re-form, but this can be avoided by making the required steering movement using the angulation controls.
- *Forceful angulation is ineffective*. With one angulation control fully angulated, applying the other control wheel only swivels the bending section very little, and scarcely affects the degree of angulation (Fig 6.22). On problem bends, therefore, concentrate on torque steering, because overforceful use of the lateral angulation control is likely to stress the angulation wires without improving the view or helping insertion.

Sigmoidoscopy—accurate steering

The sigmoid colon is an elastic tube (Fig 6.23a). When inflated it becomes long and tortuous; when deflated it is significantly shorter. When stretched by a colonoscope, especially if overinflated as well, the bowel inevitably forms both loops and acute bends (Fig 6.23b). However, it can also be shortened back, deflated, and telescoped into a few convoluted centimeters over the colonoscope (Fig 6.23c), just as a rolled-up shirt sleeve crumples over the arm.
- *Suction air frequently and fluid infrequently*. A perfect view is not necessary during insertion. Whenever fully distended colon is seen or the patient feels discomfort, suction out excess gas until the colon outline starts to wrinkle and collapse, making it shorter and easier to manipulate. Having evacuated fluid from the rectum, for the rest of the insertion phase only aspirate fluid when absolutely necessary to

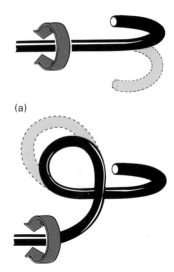

(a)

(b)

Fig 6.21 (a) Twist only affects the tip if the shaft is straight, (b) but it only affects the loop if one is present.

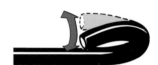

Fig 6.22 Lateral control angulation has little effect if the tip is maximally up- or down-angulated.

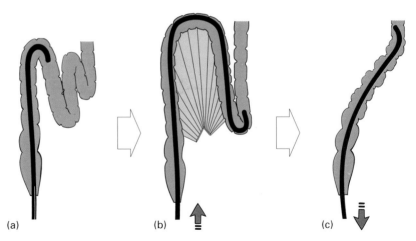

Fig 6.23 (a) The sigmoid colon is an elastic tube; (b) pushing loops it (c) but pulling back shortens and straightens the colon.

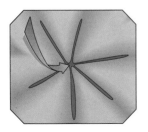

Fig 6.24 Aim at the convergence of folds, muscle fibers, or reflected highlights.

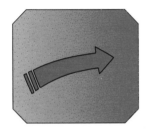

Fig 6.25 Aim at the darkest area.

keep a view. During insertion there will be numerous local "sumps" or pools of residual fluid; aspirating each one wastes time, loses the view, and requires reinflation. It is often better to inflate a little before suctioning, because suctioning blindly under fluid is often rather ineffectual and tends to lead to mucosal "suction blebs." It is quite appropriate to steer in over fluid levels during insertion, because the residual fluid can more easily be suctioned or removed by position change during withdrawal, when a perfect view is essential.

• *Insufflate as little as possible*. A distended colon is less manageable and more uncomfortable than a nondistended one. Gentle insufflation is needed throughout the examination to keep a view. However, the policy for inflation is "as much as necessary, as little as possible"; it is essential to see the colon but counterproductive to overdistend it.

• *Bubbles should be avoided or removed*. They are caused by insufflating under water (angulate above it before insufflating, see Fig 6.14) or by the detergent action of bile salts. Bubbles affect the accuracy of view but can be dispersed instantly by syringe-flushing 20 mL silicone emulsion anti-bubble solution down the instrument channel, followed by 20 mL air to clear the channel. Preparations used to avoid wind in babies are suitable for this purpose.

• *Use all visual clues*. A perfect view is not essential for progress but the endoscopist should be as sure as possible about the correct direction or axis of the colonic lumen, ascertained before pushing in. With only a partial or close-up view of the mucosal surface, there are usually sufficient clues to detect the luminal direction (Video 6.6):

– the lumen (when deflated or in spasm) is at the center of converging folds (Fig 6.24);

– aim toward the darkest (worst illuminated) area because it is furthest from the instrument and nearest the lumen (Fig 6.25);

– the convex arcs formed by haustral folds or the wrinkling of circular muscles and indicate the center of the arc, so the correct direction in which to steer (Fig 6.26);

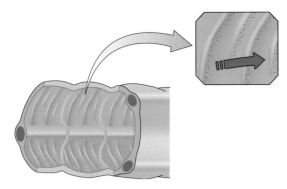

Fig 6.26 Aim at the center of the arc formed by folds.

– in a capacious colon the muscle bulk of a tenia coli (Fig 6.27) can show as a longitudinal fold which, helpfully, follows the direction of the lumen.

- *Torque-steer, single-handed and cerebrally.* Each bend requires a conscious steering decision, but by combining up/down angulation and finger-grip rotation of the shaft, much of the sigmoid can be rapidly traversed with little or no use of the lateral angulation control. The angulated tip "corkscrews" efficiently, first one way and then the other, round the succession of bends.

- *Concentrate on the monitor view* and suppress the normal social reflexes of looking at the patient or colleagues when talking to them. Acute bends or small polyps may disappear from view as the endoscopist looks away, and can take a surprisingly long time to find again.

- *Rehearse steering actions* before bends, while there is a "good" view. The give-away of a really acute bend may only be a bright angular fold seen against a darker background (Fig 6.28). Unlike the stomach, where there is usually sufficient room to see what is happening during steering maneuvers, colonic bends can be unforgivingly tight, so it is very easy to become unsighted and uncertain when angling around them. It is often best to stop before an acute bend and try out, while stationary and still able to see, the best steering movements to use once impacted within it. "Pre-steering" allows the scope to enter an acute bend at a mechanical advantage (Fig 6.29).

- *If there is no view, pull back at once.* Pushing blindly, especially if there is a "red out" and total loss of view, is usually a pointless waste of time, and potentially a cause of perforation. If lost at any point in the examination, keep the angulation controls still or let them go entirely, then insufflate and gently withdraw the instrument until the mucosa and its vessel pattern slips slowly past the lens in a proximal direction (Fig 6.30, Video 6.6). Steer towards the direction of slippage by angulating the controls or twisting the shaft, and the lumen of the colon should come back into view. Thrashing around blindly with the instrument rarely works; pulling back must help, for the bending section self-straightens if left free to do so. An expert "lost" for more than 5–10 seconds will admit it and pull back quickly to regain the view and re-orientate; the beginner flounders around in each difficult spot and is then surprised that the overall examination has taken so long.

Fig 6.27 At acute bends a longitudinal bulge (tenia coli) shows the axis to follow.

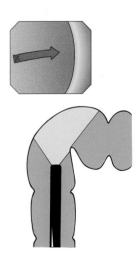

Fig 6.28 Endoscopic view of an acute bend, with a bright fold on the angle, and the "aerial" view.

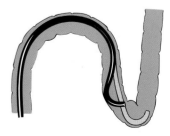

Fig 6.29 Pre-steer before pushing into an acute bend.

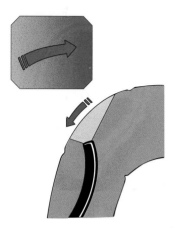

Fig 6.30 Pull back when lost—the mucosa slides away in the direction of the lumen.

• *Blind "slide-by" over the mucosa is occasionally permissible*, but only if unavoidable, for a few seconds and a few centimeters. The scope should slip easily over the surface, with the "slide-by" appearance of mucosal vascular pattern traversing the field of view. Only push on if this "slide-by" continues smoothly. If progress stops or causes the patient pain, stop at once, pull back and try again. Force alone is rarely the answer during colonoscopy.

• *Try position change*. Changing the patient from side to the back or right side not only lets gravity reposition fluid and gas, but also moves the colon, often with surprisingly beneficial results. A loop or bend that seems awkward or impassable with the patient in one position often becomes dramatically easier after position change.

Endoscopic anatomy of the sigmoid and descending colon

The sigmoid colon is 50–70 cm or more in length when stretched by the instrument during insertion, although it will crumple down to only 30–35 cm when the instrument is straightened fully, which is why careful inspection is important during insertion if lesions are not to be missed during the withdrawal phase. The sigmoid colon mesentery is inserted in a V-shape across the pelvic brim, but is very variable in both insertion and length, and also quite frequently modified by adhesions from previous inflammatory disease or surgery. After hysterectomy the distal sigmoid colon can be angulated and fixed anteriorly into the space vacated by the uterus.

The colonoscope may stretch the bowel to the limits of its attachments or the confines of the abdominal cavity. The shape of the pelvis, with its curved sacral hollow and the forward-projecting sacral promontory, cause the colonoscope to pass anteriorly (Fig 6.31a) so that the shaft can often be felt looped onto the anterior abdominal wall before it passes posteriorly again to the descending colon in the left paravertebral gutter (Fig 6.31b). The result is that

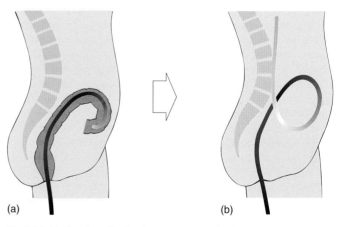

(a)   (b)

Fig 6.31 (a) The sigmoid colon loops anteriorly, (b) then passes up into the left paravertebral gutter.

an anteroposterior loop occurs during passage of the sigmoid colon and, since the descending colon is usually laterally placed, it tends to form a clockwise spiral loop (Fig 6.32, Video 6.7); the importance of this will be discussed later. When the sigmoid loop runs anteriorly against the abdominal wall it is possible partially to reduce or modify the sigmoid looping of the colonoscope by pressing against the left lower abdomen with the hand (Fig 6.33).

The descending colon is normally bound down retroperitoneally, so ideally runs in a fixed straight line, which is easy to pass with the colonoscope, except that there is usually an iatrogenic acute bend at the junction with the sigmoid colon (Fig 6.34). This junction is only a theoretical landmark to the radiologist but, once the sigmoid colon is deformed upwards by the colonoscope shaft, the resulting angulation becomes a very real challenge to the endoscopist. The acuteness of the sigmoid–descending angle depends on anatomical factors, including how far down in the pelvis the descending colon is fixed, but also on colonoscopic insertion technique. A really acute hairpin bend results when the sigmoid colon is long or elastic enough to make a large loop, and retroperitoneal fixation of the descending colon happens also to be low in the pelvis (Fig 6.35). Sometimes, when the sigmoid colon is long, an "alpha" spiral loop occurs, blessedly for both endoscopist and patient, which avoids any angulation at the sigmoid–descending junction. The "alpha" describes the shape of the spiral loop of sigmoid colon twisted around on its mesentery or sigmoid mesocolon into a partial iatrogenic volvulus (Fig 6.36). Formation of the loop depends on the anatomical fact that the short inverted "V" base of the sigmoid mesocolon twists easily, providing that the sigmoid is long enough, there are no adhesions, and the descending colon is conventionally fixed.

Mesenteric fixation variations occur because of partial or complete failure of retroperitoneal fixation of the descending colon in utero. The result is persistence of varying degrees of descending mesocolon, which in turn has a considerable effect on what shape the

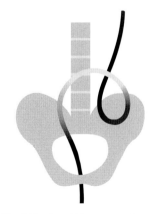

Fig 6.32 Sigmoid loop—anterior view (clockwise spiral).

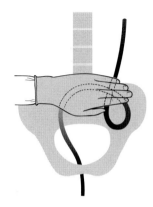

Fig 6.33 Hand-pressure restricts the sigmoid spiral loop.

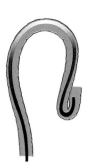

Fig 6.34 Fixed (iatrogenic) hairpin bend at the sigmoid-descending colon junction.

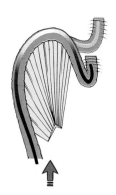

Fig 6.35 The length of the mesentery and the extent of retroperitoneal fixation determine the acuteness of the sigmoid–descending junction.

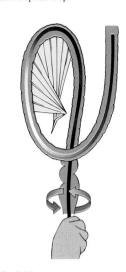

Fig 6.36 An alpha loop—a beneficial iatrogenic volvulus.

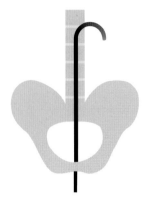

Fig 6.37 The endoscope may push a fully mobile distal colon up the midline to the diaphragm.

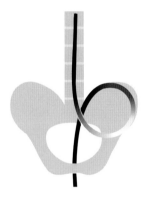

Fig 6.38 A reversed alpha loop due to a persistent descending mesocolon.

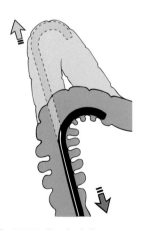

Fig 6.39 Pulling back flattens out an acute bend and improves the view.

colonoscope can force the colon into during insertion. The descending colon can, for instance, run up the midline (Fig 6.37) or allow a "reversed alpha" loop to form (Fig 6.38). Surgeons are well aware that there is great patient-to-patient variation in how easily the colon can be mobilized and delivered outside the abdominal cavity; occasionally the whole colon can be lifted out without dissection. A colon that is "easy" for the surgeon to mobilize is, however, often extremely unpredictable and "difficult" for endoscope insertion, because it is so mobile and pushes into atypical loops.

Sigmoidoscopy—the bends

Colons also vary greatly in elasticity and pain sensitivity—the sigmoid colon particularly. A degree of looping that is well tolerated by one patient may be unacceptably traumatic for another. The most challenging part of colonoscopy is to traverse the sigmoid as safely, gently, and rapidly as feasible. How best to achieve this depends on the anatomy and physiology of the individual patient, finessed by the equipment chosen and the endoscopist's handskills and judgment.

Shorten acute or mobile bends by pulling back. Having angled around an acute bend, if the view is poor, gently pull back the hooked scope, which should simultaneously reduce the angle, shorten the bowel distally, straighten it out proximally, and dis-impact the tip to give a better view (Fig 6.39). Because the colon can rotate on its attachments, bends may change during such maneuvering, any rotation being visible in close-up as a rotation of the visible vessel pattern (Fig 6.40). Watch the vessel pattern rotation carefully in close-up to know which direction to follow if a mobile bend rotates when pushing or pulling it.

The colonoscope will pass an acute bend more easily if:
• *the bend axis is oriented upward or downward* (easiest for thumb angulation)
• *the shaft is straight* (for more effective push)
• *the bowel is deflated slightly*
• *the bending section is not over-angulated* (to help it slide around).

Over-angulation, using both controls, tends to wedge the scope into a bend, making it unlikely to slide around. In the quest to get a better view around a difficult bend it is easy to forget this unproductive "walking-stick handle" effect (Fig 6.41).

Seeing the lumen doesn't always mean that it's safe to push. The acute angulation possible with modern endoscopes (see Fig 6.23b) can mislead the endoscopist, giving a spuriously good view ahead when the bending section is jack-knifed and hopelessly impacted into an acute bend (such as the sigmoid–descending junction).

If in doubt . . . pull out.

Sigmoidoscopy—the loops

Colons vary hugely in length and attachments, with further constraints from surrounding organs and the limits of the abdominal cavity or any adhesions. Young men mostly have a short colon, unless constipated or with hemorrhoids. Women tend to have a longer colon, especially those with constipation. Longer colons allow more looping, but are often relatively pain insensitive (partly because the colon moves so easily), so the patient may suffer less than the endoscopist.

Sigmoid looping of some degree is unavoidable as the scope pushes up the apex of the sigmoid colon (Video 6.8).

Clues suggesting a loop has formed are:
• *loss of "one-to-one" relationship* between the amount of shaft being inserted through the anus and the movement inwards of the scope tip;
• *"wind pain"* is the commonest warning of looping, and only acceptable providing that the discomfort is mild and the scope tip is advancing rapidly;
• *"paradoxical movement,"* in which the instrument tip slides outward as the shaft is pushed in (or vice versa), which suggests a substantial loop;
• *the angulation controls feel "jammed up."* As the scope loops, increasing friction in the wires from the angulation controls to the bending section causes the controls to feel stiffer and stiffer, but with less and less steering effect.

Inexperienced endoscopists often do not notice these clues, can become deaf to patient protest (or overgenerous with sedation), and think that forceful management of the colonoscope is "normal." Colonoscopy should (mostly) be a deft and gentle procedure, manageable by finger-grip and fine movements.

Instrument stretch pressure into a loop feels like "wind" or the "urge to go." The patient should be warned before using force and whenever push begins to cause looping or discomfort (e.g. "you will feel some wind pain for a few seconds, but there is no danger"). Uncomfortable push should be limited to a tolerable time—ideally no more than 20–30 seconds. Looping pain stops at once when the instrument is withdrawn slightly, so there is no excuse for long-continued periods of pain, even in examinations where recurrent loops form.

Abdominal hand-pressure can be helpful, but only when the sigmoid happens to loop anteriorly, close to the abdominal wall (Fig 6.31), which is especially likely in a protuberant abdomen or "beer belly." The assistant compressing nonspecifically over the lower abdomen, which opposes the sigmoid loop, may reduce stretch pain and can make the scope slide around more easily. Assistant hand-pressure is only relevant during the 20–30 seconds needed to resist looping during inward scope-push. There is no need to fatigue the assistant by asking for more prolonged hand-pressure, especially as in around 50% of patients the sigmoid loop is nowhere near the abdominal surface.

Gentle "push through" the sigmoid colon is allowable, providing it is easy and requires no undue force. Using careful steering combined with "persuasive pressure" the scope may slide around the bends of the sigmoid and up into the descending colon (Fig 6.42).

Inward push should be applied gradually, avoiding sudden thrusts. Shorter sigmoid loops require more subtlety and often

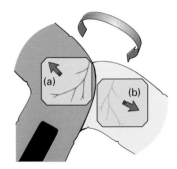

Fig 6.40 Rotation of the vessel pattern (from (a) to (b)) indicates rotation of the colon, so the endoscopist needs to change steering direction too.

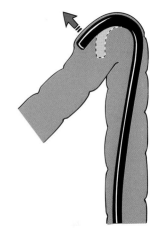

Fig 6.41 De-angulate at the splenic flexure to avoid "walking-stick handle" impaction.

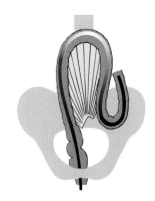

Fig 6.42 A very long sigmoid may allow the scope to "push though" and avoid forming a hairpin bend.

cause more pain, as their short mesenteric attachments are restrictive and stretch force is more localized and obvious. Pushing is most likely to be effective in a longer colon, which tends to accommodate to the instrument, letting it slide in more freely with no acute bends and more likelihood of favorable (spiral) loops.

It is dangerous to ignore pain (or suppress it with heavy sedation or anesthesia) and to push into a loop when the scope tip is jammed and not progressing.

Short or pain-sensitive colons—pull back and straighten the "N"-loop

Although some degree of looping is inevitable as the instrument pushes inward, in a short colon the endoscopist may, by subtlety, repeatedly pulling back, avoiding insufflation, and deflating whenever possible, be able to achieve virtually "direct" passage from sigmoid to descending colon with minimal stretch (Fig 6.43). This is elegant technically and comfortable for the patient.

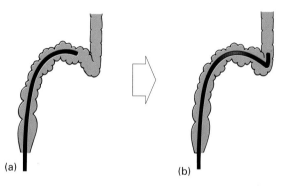

(a)   (b)

Fig 6.43 (a) Pull back and deflate to keep the sigmoid short, (b) which may allow direct passage to the descending colon.

Upward "N"-looping of a short colon is the classic loop of colonoscopy. "N"-looping causes the scope tip to approach the sigmoid–descending junction at an acute angle or hairpin bend (Fig 6.44), but this can potentially be straightened back so that the instrument is able to slide directly (and painlessly) up the descending colon (Video 6.9).

At the sigmoid–descending junction the scope enters retroperitoneal fixation, so it is a good place to try to pull back and get control of the sigmoid loop while the tip and bending section are fixed. Direct passage straight up the descending colon is the ideal, trying to steer the tip around the junction without forcing up the sigmoid loop. This takes subtlety, and even experts can have trouble in achieving it, pulling back, twisting, and steering cautiously (usually with a poor view). Typically a less skilled endoscopist, having slid around the sigmoid with panache, will have stretched up a large (iatrogenic) sigmoid loop (Fig 6.45a) and so created an acute hairpin bend (and extra difficulty) as a result. Being more careful, using less air, less push, and then pulling back vigorously (Fig 6.45b) can be rewarded by "direct" passage from the sigmoid to descending colon (Fig 6.45c).

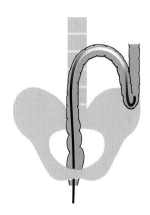

Fig 6.44 An "N"-loop stretching up the sigmoid colon.

There can be a useful "N-spiral" element because most sigmoid loops run in a clockwise spiral—anteriorly out of the pelvis, over the pelvic brim, then curving laterally and posteriorly into the descending colon (see Fig 6.31). The resulting spiral shape can be used by a single-handed endoscopist to corkscrew directly around (with strong clockwise shaft twist) into the descending colon, with a minimum of push force, and so no re-looping (Fig 6.46, Video 6.9).

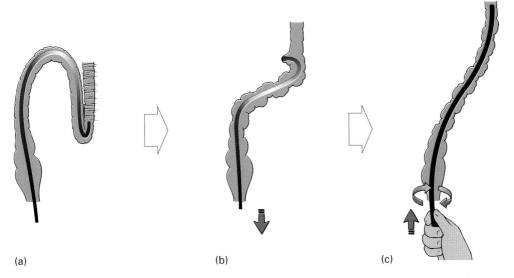

(a)   (b)   (c)

Fig 6.45 (a) The tip is hooked into the retroperitoneal descending colon, then pulled back, (b) and when the endoscope is maximally straightened (sometimes "blind") the tip is redirected (c) and the endoscope pushed in, usually with clockwise twist, up the descending colon.

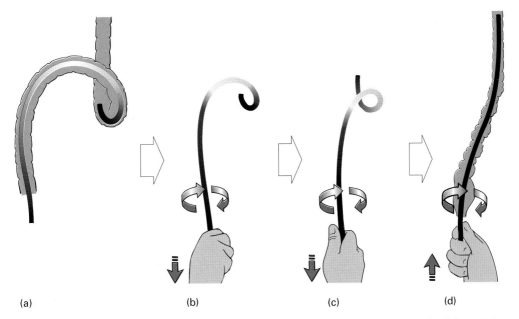

(a)   (b)   (c)   (d)

Fig 6.46 (a) An "N"-loop with the tip at the sigmoid–descending junction, (b) twist clockwise and withdraw, (c) keep twisting and find the lumen of the descending colon, (d) then push in (still twisting forcibly to prevent re-looping).

A pain-sensitive colon suggests trying this "short-scope" "N-spiral" approach. Pulling back and deflating during insertion around the sigmoid and taking extra care (and time) to withdraw, twisting clockwise and trying to straighten at the sigmoid–descending junction (see below) will often achieve direct painless passage into the descending colon. This largely explains why the technique of some endoscopists allows them to perform successful colonoscopy with little or no sedation while others routinely rely on heavy sedation or anesthesia.

At the sigmoid–descending junction try the following steps.

1 *Pull back the shaft* to reduce the loop, which creates a more favorable angle of approach to the junction and also optimizes the instrument mechanics (see Fig 6.43).

2 *Deflate* (without losing the view) to shorten the colon and make it as pliable as possible.

3 *Apply abdominal pressure*. The assistant pushes on the left lower abdomen so as to compress the loop or reduce the abdominal space.

4 *Pull back with shaft twist* in the hope that corkscrewing force will direct the angulated tip into the descending colon and hold it there (see Fig 6.46). Successful "pull-with-clockwise-twist" uses this tip fixation, together with scope withdrawal, to shorten ("pleat," "accordion," "concertina") the sigmoid over the colonoscope shaft, while simultaneously sliding the tip up the descending colon. Sometimes the act of pulling causes the hooked tip to impact into the mucosa (Fig 6.45b). Careful angulation control is needed, any wrong move being likely to lose the critical retroperitoneal tip fixation and cause the instrument to fall back into the sigmoid. When the maneuver is successful (Fig 6.45c) the endoscopist has the warm feeling of "getting something for nothing," passing directly into descending colon without looping or pain.

5 *Change the patient to supine or right lateral position*. This can improve the view of the sigmoid–descending junction (air rises, water falls) and may sometimes also cause the distal descending colon to drop down into a more favorable configuration for passage.

6 *Forceful "push through" the loop should be the last option*. It may sometimes be better to warn the patient and push in calculatedly rather than struggling with repeated failed attempts at shortening. A few seconds (typically 20–30 seconds) of careful "persuasive pressure" may slide the instrument tip around the bend and then allow straightening again.

Suspect a spiral or alpha loop if insertion seems easy. If, during insertion, no particularly acute flexure is encountered in the sigmoid colon and the instrument appears to be sliding in a long way without problems or acute angulations, it is possible that a spiral or alpha loop is being formed (Video 6.10). If so (especially if confirmed on fluoroscopy or the magnetic imager) push on to the proximal descending colon or splenic flexure before trying any withdrawal/straightening maneuver. Even if the patient has mild stretch pain, reassure and continue, steering carefully until the tip has passed through the fluid-filled descending colon to the splenic flexure, reached at about 90 cm (Fig 6.47). Straightening back halfway round a spiral loop is a mistake, as this may cause the spiral alpha configuration to rotate back into N-loop configuration, which then results in greater difficulty in reaching the descending colon (alternatively, it may fall back, require reinsertion, and so prolong the uncomfortable insertion phase).

A long sigmoid colon tends to push into a spiral loop. A spiral loop can occur in around 60% of patients; in 10% the spiral is flat against the posterior abdominal wall in "alpha" shape, as originally described with the patient lying flat for x-ray fluoroscopy (Fig 6.48). Using the magnetic or 3D imager (ScopeGuide®, Olympus) allows loops to be assessed from the lateral view as well as anteroposterior view (Fig 6.49a,b, Video 6.11), showing a much greater frequency of spiral configuration. Any spiral loop is a blessing, since the shape means that there is no acute bend between the sigmoid and descending colon so that, with continued inward push (Fig 6.49c) the scope can slide relatively easily into the descending colon with no resistance, before being straightened (Fig 6.49d).

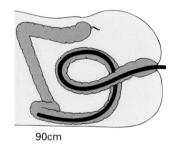

90cm

Fig 6.47 In an alpha loop the scope runs through the fluid-filled descending colon to the splenic flexure at 90 cm (posterior view—as for the endoscopist).

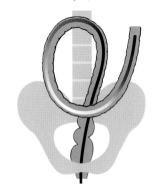

Fig 6.48 An alpha loop.

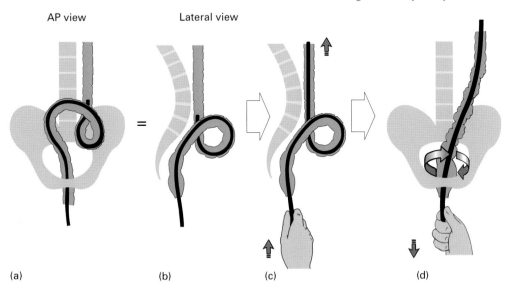

AP view   Lateral view

(a)   (b)   (c)   (d)

Fig 6.49 Many "N"-loops (a), if also seen in lateral view (b) are actually spiral, so (c) push on toward the splenic flexure before (d) straightening back.

It may take several attempts to create a spiral loop. Inserting around a long and tortuous sigmoid the endoscopist may struggle to disimpact the scope tip from several acute angulations, but the act of doing so can reposition the colon into spiral shape, with sudden improvement of view and the opportunity for successful progress. This process of (gently) bullying the colon to produce a spiral loop was historically called "the alpha maneuver" (Fig 6.50). It typically involved counterclockwise twisting force under x-ray control and helped insertion of early colonoscopes, which had limited angulation characteristics so as to protect their fragile glass-fiber bundles. The concept of encouraging spiral loop configuration, or of making the most of the opportunity when it occurs spontaneously, remains a valuable option even with modern instrumentation (especially if the magnetic imager is available for guidance).

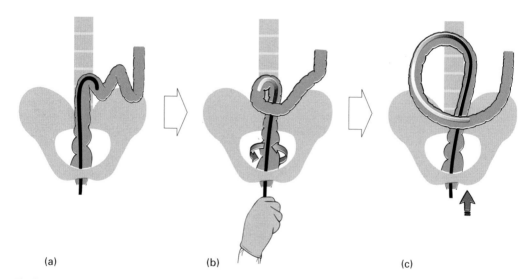

(a)   (b)   (c)

Fig 6.50 "The alpha maneuver": During sigmoidal insertion, (b) try counterclockwise rotation to point the tip toward the cecum; (c) and push in to form an alpha or spiral loop.

Straightening a spiral loop

A spiral or alpha loop must be removed at some stage, usually before pushing around the splenic flexure, to avoid stressing the patient and scope. Most colonoscopists prefer to straighten out the loop (to 50 cm) as soon as the upper descending colon or splenic flexure is safely reached (at 90 cm) and then to pass around the flexure with a straightened instrument. However, every colonoscopist has also experienced the chagrin of seeing the tip slide back when a straightening attempt is made too early, before the tip is adequately fixed by friction or angulation. It can occasionally be better in an unusually long but mobile colon to pass around the splenic flexure into the transverse colon with the spiral loop still in place.

Spiral loop straightening is simply an exaggerated version of the "pull back and twist" maneuver described above, combining a withdrawal with strong clockwise rotation to remove the loop in a few seconds (Fig 6.51, Videos 6.7–6.11). Withdrawing the shaft initially reduces the size of the loop and makes de-rotational twisting easier. Twist alone would change the sigmoid spiral into an "N" shape but not straighten the loop. By combining the two actions, simultaneously and rapidly pulling back and twisting the whole instrument, the loop is smoothly and easily removed to 50–60 cm, often in only 2–3 seconds and with obvious improvement of the "feel" as the shaft straightens (see Fig 6.46). The clockwise twist used should push the tip inward towards the splenic flexure. Any tendency to slip back is prevented by applying more twist and less pull, or by hooking the tip more actively into the splenic flexure. Such twisting forces do not harm the colonoscope.

De-rotation should be easy and atraumatic. If straightening the loop proves difficult or the patient has discomfort, the situation, should be reassessed. Do not use excessive force. The sigmoid loop that has formed may not be a clockwise spiral loop but a "reversed alpha" (see below). In the absence of magnetic imager, the endoscopist must judge this by feel (and results).

Longer colons—the S-loop

When "pushing-through" a very long sigmoid colon, a flat S-shaped loop may form, with no spiral configuration (Video 6.12)—so twist has no effect when pulling back to straighten it. The key to success is to push on to the splenic flexure, angulating around it to fix the tip before removing the loop. **Pulling back before the tip is properly angulated usually allows the scope to slip back, which means having reintroduce around the bend (easier to assess using a magnetic imager).**

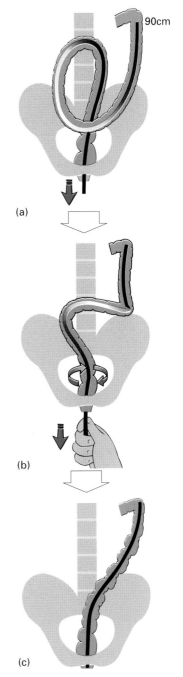

(a)

(b)

(c)

Fig 6.51 (a) An alpha loop (b) de-rotates with clockwise twist and withdrawal (c) to straighten completely.

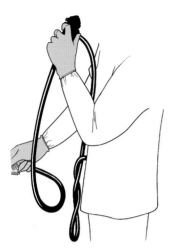

Fig 6.52 Shaft loops forming outside the patient can be transferred to the umbilical by rotating the control body.

Atypical sigmoid loops and the "reversed alpha"

"Atypical" spiral loops can form when colon attachments are unusually mobile, particularly those of the descending colon (see below). The colonoscope may force a mobile colon into an counterclockwise spiral, or even a complex mix of clockwise and counterclockwise loops. In practical terms this variation should make little difference to the endoscopist, except for the need to apply the correct de-rotational force when pulling back to straighten. A counterclockwise "reversed alpha" loop (see Fig 6.38) may allow the scope tip to slide up into the descending colon as easily as a conventional spiral loop, with no obvious clue that there is anything odd or unusual. As around 90% of sigmoid loops spiral clockwise, the unsuspecting endoscopist can waste time and make things worse by trying to derotate the atypical (counterclockwise) loop with conventional clockwise twist. If a magnetic imager is being used, the configuration and its solution are obvious. If relying on shaft feel and guesswork, try counterclockwise twist if the sigmoid appears not to be straightening. Occasionally de-rotational twist has to be first one way, then the other.

Remove shaft loops external to the patient

Straightening colonic loops may result in shaft loops external to the patient. The mechanical construction of an endoscope, with its protective wire claddings and four angulation wires, means that any shaft loop increases the resistance of the instrument to twisting/torquing movements. Looping also decreases tip angulation by causing friction in the angulation wires. For this reason shaft loops are mechanically undesirable even when they occur outside the patient. The shaft should run in an easy curve to the anus, without unnecessary bends. Any loops forming outside the patient should ideally be derotated and straightened. This is easily done by rotating the control body to transfer the loop to the umbilical (which can accommodate up to three loops without harm to its internal structures) (Fig 6.52). Sometimes it may be necessary to unplug the light guide connector from the light source and then unravel the umbilical. The alternative for the dexterous endoscopist is to derotate the external shaft loop by twist, while steering the tip into the lumen, the straightened colonoscope rotating on its axis.

Diverticular disease

In severe diverticular disease there may be a narrowed lumen, pericolic adhesions, and problems in choosing the correct direction (Fig 6.53a). However, once the instrument has been laboriously inched through the area, the "splinting" effect of the abnormally rigid sigmoid may facilitate the rest of the examination by preventing any sigmoid loop from re-forming. The secret in diverticular disease is extreme patience, with care in visualization and steering combined with greater than usual use of withdrawal, rotatory, or corkscrewing movements. It helps to realize that a close-up view of a diverticulum means that the tip is at right angles to the lumen

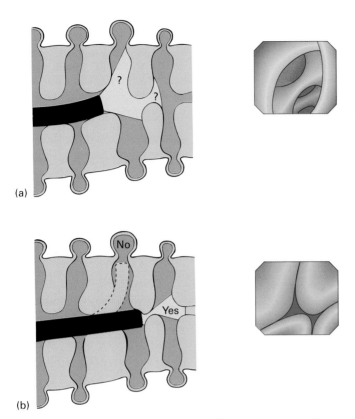

Fig 6.53 (a) Choosing the correct path can be difficult in diverticular disease: (b) a circular view is a diverticulum—the lumen will be at 90°, and often squashed.

and must be deflected or withdrawn to find the lumen, which is often deformed and unobvious (Fig 6.53b).

Using a thinner and more flexible pediatric colonoscope or gastroscope may make an apparently impassable narrow, fixed, or angulated sigmoid colon relatively easy to examine, which sometimes also saves the patient from surgery.

Having successfully passed severe fixed or angulated sigmoid diverticular disease (especially if it has taken a short scope to do so), it becomes the endoscopist's worst nightmare if the proximal colon then proves to be long and mobile.

If the tip is fixed or impacted it cannot be steered. The tip and bending section of a flexible endoscope normally angulates because it is free to move easily. If the tip is fixed, attempted angulation simply moves the shaft around instead (Fig 6.54). This is an inherent limiting factor of flexible endoscopes, and is why the endoscopist may be unable to steer effectively in fixed diverticular disease or to get a proper view in a tight stricture. Torque is less affected in such situations, which is another reason why torque-steering is so useful.

"Underwater colonoscopy" may help passage in some patients with very hypertrophic musculature and redundant mucosal folds,

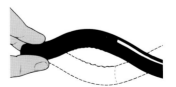

Fig 6.54 If the tip is flexed it cannot be steered (the shaft moves instead).

in whom it can be difficult to obtain an adequate view. Water can distend a narrow segment better than air, having the combined advantages of being noncompressible, remaining in the dependent sigmoid colon (rather than the tendency of air to rise and distend only the proximal colon), and holding the mucosal folds away from the lens for an improved close-up view. Except in these circumstances or to improve the close-up view in a stricture diverticulosis, it is our experience that underwater colonoscopy has nothing to offer the endoscopist compared to conventional insufflation coupled with patience, position change, and the maneuvers described above.

Be prepared to abandon if postoperative or diverticular adhesions have fixed the colon, making passage impossible or dangerous. If there is difficulty, if the instrument tip feels fixed and cannot be moved by angling or twisting and the patient complains of pain during attempts at insertion, there is a danger of perforation, and the attempt should be abandoned. Sometimes a different endoscope (e.g. pediatric colonoscope or gastroscope) or another endoscopist may succeed. Only a very experienced colonoscopist with very good clinical reasons should put the patient and instrument at risk under these circumstances; usually the most experienced are the most prepared to stop and refer for CT colography.

Descending colon

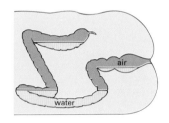

Fig 6.55 Fluid levels in the left lateral position.

The descending colon can be a 20-cm-long "straight," traversed in a few seconds. For the gravitational reasons described above, when the patient is in the left lateral position there is characteristically a horizontal fluid level (Fig 6.55, Video 6.13). Often there is sufficient air interface above the descending colon fluid (or blood in emergency cases) to allow the scope to be steered above it. If fluid makes steering difficult, it may be quicker, rather than wasting time suctioning and reinflating, to turn the patient onto his or her back or right side to fill the descending colon with air. Apart from this positional trick, and the frequent use of clockwise twist or hand-pressure to minimize sigmoid colon re-looping, no particular skills or maneuvers are needed in the average descending colon. In a long colon the descending may be so tortuous that the endoscopist, having struggled through a number of bends and fluid-filled sumps, believes the scope has arrived in the proximal colon when it has only reached the splenic flexure.

Distal colon mobility and "reversed" looping

If the descending colon is mobile, without retroperitoneal fixation, the normal anatomy can disappear. At the most extreme, the colonoscope may run through the "sigmoid" and "descending" distal colon straight up the midline (see Fig 6.37), inevitably resulting in a "reversed splenic flexure" and consequent mechanical problems later in the examination. The endoscopist is alerted to this when counterclockwise rotation seems to help insertion at the sigmoid–descending junction. This indicates that an unconventional counterclockwise spiral loop or "reversed alpha" has been formed by the instrument (see Fig 6.38), with the corollary that other oddities may occur during insertion. The endoscopist can use counterclockwise twist to push the mobile descending colon outward against the lateral margin of the abdominal cavity. This regains the conventional configuration so that the instrument runs medially (rather than in reverse) around the splenic flexure, and is able to adopt the favorable "question-mark" shape to reach the cecum. Such apparently mysterious manipulations become understandable under fluoroscopic control or with the ScopeGuide® magnetic imager.

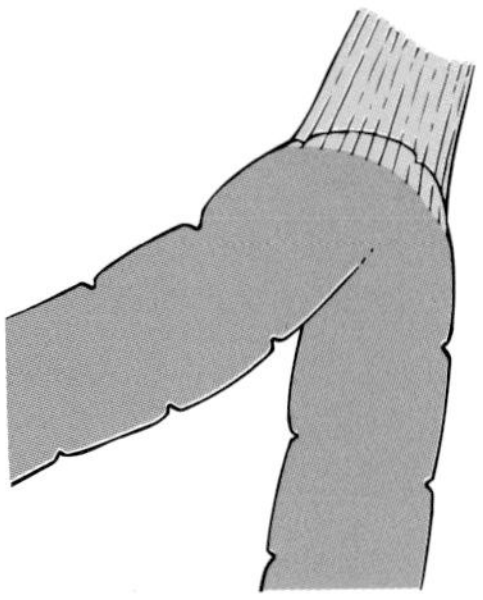

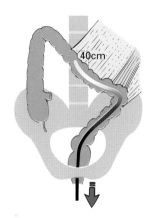

Fig 6.56 The phrenicocolic ligament.

Splenic flexure

Endoscopic anatomy

The splenic flexure is where the colon angulates medially and anteriorly beneath the left costal margin, inaccessible to hand-pressure. The position of the flexure is variably fixed according to the degree of mobility of the fold of peritoneum—the phrenicocolic ligament—which attaches it to the diaphragmatic surface (Fig 6.56). In some subjects the splenic flexure is tethered high up into the left hypochondrium, but in others it is relatively free and can be pulled down toward the pelvis (Fig 6.57). A lax phrenicocolic ligament, a common feature of long, mobile colons, makes control of the transverse colon more difficult by depriving the endoscopist of any fixed point or fulcrum with which to exert leverage during withdrawal maneuvers (the cantilever effect). The configuration of the splenic flexure is also affected by the patient's position, principally because of the effects on it of the transverse colon, which sags down under gravity in the left lateral position (Fig 6.58a) or pulls it open in the right lateral position (Fig 6.58b).

Fig 6.57 The splenic flexure can pull back to 40 cm if there is a free phrenicocolic ligament.

Insertion around the splenic flexure

The splenic flexure is the "half-time" point of colonoscopy, where the instrument should straighten back to 50 cm from the anus. This ensures that the colonoscope is under proper control before tackling the proximal colon. The commonest reason for experiencing problems in the proximal colon is because the colonoscope has

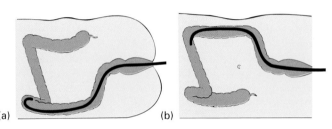

(a)   (b)

Fig 6.58 (a) In the left lateral position the transverse colon flops down, making the splenic flexure acute, (b) whereas in the right lateral position (or supine) gravity rounds off the flexure and makes it easier to pass.

been inadequately straightened at the splenic flexure. Persistence of loops makes the rest of the procedure progressively more difficult or impossible. If the splenic flexure is passed with straight shaft configuration (at 50 cm), using the above rules, the rest of colonoscopy insertion should usually be finished within a minute or two.

Anyone who frequently finds the proximal colon or hepatic flexure difficult to traverse should apply the "50 cm rule" at the splenic flexure, and is likely to find most of the problem solved, because the distal colon has been properly straightened.

Passage around the apex of the splenic flexure is usually obvious when the instrument emerges from fluid into the air-filled, often triangular, transverse colon (Fig 6.59). However, while the flexible and angulated bending section of the colonoscope passes around without effort, the stiffer segment at around 10–15 cm in the leading part of the shaft does not follow so easily. This problem is accentuated in the left lateral position, because drooping of the transverse colon causes the splenic flexure to be acutely angled (see Fig 6.58a) compared with its configuration when opened out by gravity in the supine or right lateral position (see Fig 6.58b).

To pass the splenic flexure without force or re-looping (**Video 6.14**):

1 *Straighten the scope.* Pull back with the tip hooked around the flexure until the instrument is around 50 cm from the anus (the distance can be 40–60 cm according to mobility of the flexure or angulation around it). This both straightens any sigmoid loop, pulls down the flexure, and rounds it off *(NB splenic avulsions or capsular tears have been reported, so be gentle).*

2 *If a variable stiffness scope is being used, stiffen it.* Once the splenic flexure is reached and the instrument is straightened, stiffen the shaft (the effect starts 30 cm from the tip, the leading part remaining flexible) to stop the sigmoid region re-looping and help inward push to slide the tip around the flexure. Once the leading part of the shaft is safely into the transverse colon, however, *unstiffen* the instrument again to allow the rest of the shaft to slide around the flexure more easily.

3 *Avoid over-angulation of the tip.* Full "bending-section" angulation results in such acute angling that it tends to impact in the splenic flexure, preventing further insertion (the "walking-stick handle" effect). Having obtained a view of the transverse colon and pulled back, consciously de-angulate a little so that the instrument runs around the outside of the bend (see Fig 6.41), even if this means worsening the view somewhat.

4 *Deflate the colon* slightly to shorten the flexure and make it malleable.

5 *Apply assistant hand-pressure* over the sigmoid colon (Fig 6.60). Any resistance encountered at the splenic flexure is likely to result in stretching upward of the sigmoid colon into an "N"-loop or spiral loop, which dissipates more and more of the inward force applied to the shaft if the loop increases. It is immediately obvious to the single-handed endoscopist that such a loop is forming, because the "one-to-one" relationship between insertion and tip progress is lost; in other words, the shaft is being pushed in but the tip moves

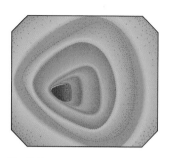

Fig 6.59 The transverse colon is usually triangular.

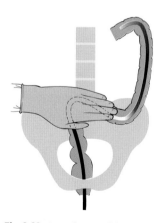

Fig 6.60 Control sigmoid looping by hand-pressure to help pass the splenic flexure.

little or not at all. Pull back again to restraighten the shaft if this occurs.

6 *Use clockwise torque on the shaft*. As explained above, the clockwise spiral course of the sigmoid colon from the pelvis to its point of fixation in the descending colon means that applying clockwise torque to the colonoscope shaft tends to counteract any looping tendency in the sigmoid colon while pushing in (Fig 6.61). Clockwise torque will only be effective to keep the shaft straight if any significant looping has first been removed by pulling back, and if the descending colon is normally fixed. Because the tip is angulated, applying clockwise shaft torque may affect the luminal view into the transverse colon, and readjustment of the angulation controls may be needed to redirect the tip.

7 *Push in, but slowly*. The instrument tip cannot advance around the splenic flexure without some degree of inward push. So, as well as clockwise twist, continued gentle inward pressure is needed (aggressive pushing simply re-forms the sigmoid loop). All that is needed for success is firm inward pressure on the shaft, which causes very gradual inward slippage of the tip into the transverse colon. While pushing, deflate again, and make any necessary compensatory steering movements. A combination of these various maneuvers, together or in sequence, using the angulation controls to "squirm" the bending section and the suction valve to collapse the bowel, may help the tip slide around the splenic flexure.

8 *If it does not work, pull back and start again*. If the tip is not progressing but from the amount of shaft being inserted it is obvious that a sigmoid loop is re-forming, pull back and run through all the above actions again before pushing in once more. It may take two or three attempts to achieve success.

9 *If it still does not work, change patient position and try again*. As pointed out earlier, the left lateral position used by most endoscopists has the undesirable effect of causing the transverse colon to flop down (see Fig 6.58a) and make the splenic flexure acutely angled. Turning the patient onto his or her back or right side has the opposite effect. The transverse colon sags to the right side and, together with gravity, often pulls the splenic flexure into a smooth curve without any apparent "flexure" at all (see Fig 6.58b).

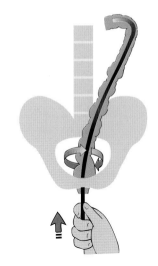

Fig 6.61 Twist the shaft clockwise while advancing to keep the sigmoid straight.

Summary: passing the splenic flexure (Video 6.14)
1 *Pull back to straighten the scope* (to around 50 cm)
2 *Stiffen a variable scope*
3 *Avoid over-angulation of the tip*
4 *Deflate the colon*
5 *Apply assistant hand-pressure*
6 *Use clockwise torque on the shaft*
7 *Push in, but slowly*
8 *If it does not work, pull back and start again*
9 *Then change position to back or right side and try again!*

Position change

Change of position does take a few seconds to achieve, and the patient has to be returned to the left lateral position to inflate and visualize the proximal colon properly before reaching the cecum.

Movement can be cumbersome if the patient is obese, disabled, or oversedated. We therefore change position if "stuck" at the splenic flexure for over 60 seconds or so, allowing several attempts at direct passage, first in the left lateral position, then the supine, before full rotation to the right. The ability to perform postural changes easily is an additional reason for reducing routine sedation (or avoiding it altogether when possible).

Position change can be made into a simple routine (Video 6.8):
1 change hands, to hold the instrument control body in the right hand;
2 raise the patient's lower foot with your left hand, lifting both legs;
3 slide the shaft through to the other side of the legs;
4 the patient can then turn over.
Providing the shaft is kept away from the patient's heels there is nothing to go wrong. The whole position-change maneuver takes at most 20–30 seconds in a lightly sedated patient. Subsequent position changes take less time still, for the patient understands what is required.

Overtubes

A stiffening overtube, sometimes called a "splinting device," is rarely used now, but may hold a looping sigmoid colon straight and allow easier passage into the proximal colon. As well as its use for stiffening a looping sigmoid colon, an overtube can be invaluable for exchanging colonoscopes or removing multiple polypectomy specimens.

The original extremely stiff (wire-reinforced) overtubes for colonoscopy had disadvantages that discouraged most endoscopists from using them. The tube had to be on the instrument before starting (or the endoscope completely withdrawn before putting it on), and insertion was sometimes traumatic, with perforations reported.

"Balloon colonoscopy" is the modern equivalent technique. The double-balloon approach incorporates an overtube with a balloon attached to the end, allowing the bowel to be compacted and sta-bilised and permitting easier progression of the scope. The single-balloon equivalent also involves a simple but relatively flexible overtube with a balloon-tipped enteroscope. Both approaches are reported to facilitate shortening maneuvers and successful intuba-tion of very long colons. However, using the techniques described in this chapter and a long ScopeGuide® magnetic imager colono-scope, we achieve over 99% complete colonoscopy without recourse to these additional instruments.

The "reversed" splenic flexure

Atypical passage around the splenic flexure is seen to occur in about 5% of patients if imaging is available. The instrument tip passes laterally rather than medially around the splenic flexure, because the descending colon has moved centrally on a mesocolon (Fig 6.62 Video 6.14). This is of more than academic interest because, having passed laterally round the flexure and displaced

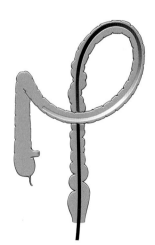

Fig 6.62 A "reversed" splenic flexure will result in a deep transverse loop.

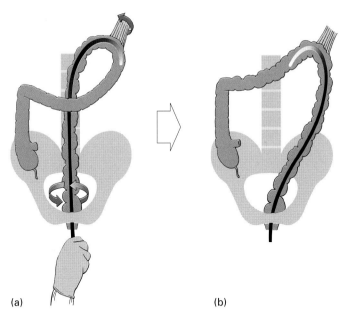

(a)   (b)

Fig 6.63 (a) Counterclockwise rotation (b) swings a mobile colon back to the normal position.

the descending colon medially, the advancing instrument forces the transverse colon down into a deep loop. The instrument is then mechanically under stress and difficult to steer, and the hepatic flexure is approached from below at a disadvantageous angle, making it difficult to reach the cecum and virtually impossible to steer into the ileo-cecal valve. With a reversed splenic loop, even when the instrument tip can be hooked onto the hepatic flexure, the sheer bulkiness of the reversed loop configuration actively holds down the transverse loop, stopping it being straightened and lifted up into the ideal "question-mark" shape.

De-rotation of a reversed splenic flexure loop may be possible and will avoid these problems later in the examination. This can be done by twisting the shaft strongly counterclockwise (rather than the usual clockwise twist), usually after withdrawing the tip toward the splenic flexure. The subsequent examination is so much quicker, and also more comfortable for the patient, that the time spent doing this can be well worthwhile. Counterclockwise de-rotation makes the tip pivot around the phrenicocolic suspensory ligament and swing medially (Fig 6.63a). After that, by maintaining counterclockwise torque while pushing in, the instrument can be made to pass across the transverse colon in the usual configuration, forcing the descending colon back laterally against the abdominal wall (Fig 6.63b).

Counterclockwise straightening is most easily performed under imaging (Video 6.14) but is also quite feasible by feel, using these guidelines and a little imagination whenever atypical looping is suspected in the proximal colon. A reversed splenic flexure/mobile descending colon is one reason for an unexpectedly difficult

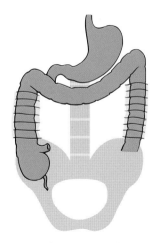

Fig 6.64 The transverse colon is anterior, over the duodenum and pancreas. The descending and ascending colon are fixed retroperitoneally.

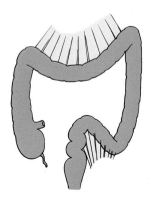

Fig 6.65 Colon mesenteries—the transverse and sigmoid mesocolons.

colonoscopy. Sometimes the best solution, if the problem is suspected but imaging is not available and attempts at counterclockwise de-rotation have failed, is simply to get a move on and to "push through" more vigorously than usual (if necessary with extra sedation) and then to abandon the procedure as soon as a reasonable view of the right colon has been obtained. For the reasons given above, if a reversed splenic loop is present, it is rare to be able to enter the ileum without successful de-rotation and straightening, because the looped and stressed instrument will not angulate sufficiently. If ileoscopy is essential and a reversed loop is present it is likely to be necessary to pull the instrument out to 50 cm at the splenic flexure, attempt counterclockwise de-rotation, and pass in again. Failing to do this and simply trying to angulate the tip forcibly into the ileum is likely to stress the bending section and not succeed.

Transverse colon

Endoscopic anatomy

In 30% of subjects the transverse colon lies anteriorly just beneath the abdominal wall, held forward by the vertebral bodies, the duodenum, and pancreas, and relates to the left and right lobes of the liver (Fig 6.64). It is enveloped in a double fold of peritoneum called the transverse mesocolon (Fig 6.65), which originates from the posterior wall of the abdomen and hangs down posterior to the stomach, varying considerably in length. In a barium enema study, the transverse colon of 62% of erect females drooped down into the pelvis, compared with only 26% of males. This longer transverse loop largely accounts for the 10–20 cm greater mean colon length found in women despite their smaller stature (total colon length was 80–180 cm) and probably also contributes to our experience that 70% of difficult colonoscopies are in women (previous hysterectomy making only a small contribution). The depth to which the transverse colon can be looped downward by colonoscope pressure also affects the angle at which the endoscope approaches the hepatic flexure, in the same way that the size of the sigmoid colon loop causes an acute sigmoid–descending colon bend. Because the transverse mesocolon (Fig 6.66a) is broad-based it is relatively unusual for a *"gamma" loop* to form (Fig 6.66b).

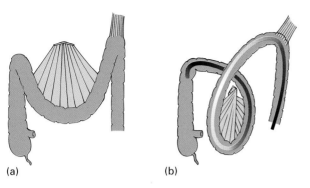

(a)   (b)

Fig 6.66 (a) Transverse mesocolon. (b) A gamma loop.

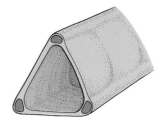

Fig 6.67 The triangular configuration is due to the three teniae coli.

The triangular configuration of the transverse colon (see Fig 6.59, Video 6.15) depends on the relative thinness of the circular muscles compared with the three longitudinal muscle bundles or teniae coli (Fig 6.67). In some patients (such as those with long-standing colitis but also some normals) the circular musculature is thicker and the transverse colon can be tubular. Both at the mid-transverse flexure and at the hepatic flexure a true "face-on" view of the haustral folds may be obtained. These present a characteristic "knife-edge" or "ladder" appearance (Fig 6.68); it is therefore easy to confuse the mid-transverse flexure with the hepatic flexure. The mid-transverse bend should be less voluminous, show no blue/gray liver patch and may show transmitted cardiac (double) or aortic (single) pulsation. It can also be distinguished by imaging, local palpation of the anterior abdominal wall or transillumination (if the room is darkened).

Insertion through the transverse colon

Insertion around the transverse should be easy, **unless** the sigmoid colon has also looped, so reducing inward force transmission. In the mid-transverse colon, however, the angled scope tip often forms a surprisingly sharp bend, pushing the loop downward into the pelvis. A drooping transverse colon, frequently found in women and those with a long colon, inevitably results in greater friction resistance to passage; the force required then results in secondary sigmoid looping as well. This combination can be a major problem for "push and go" endoscopists who have not learned the wisdom of shortening and controlling colon loops (Video 6.16).

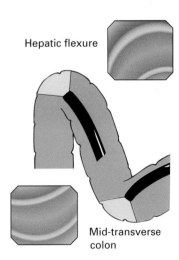

Hepatic flexure

Mid-transverse colon

Fig 6.68 Similar "knife-like" haustra are seen at the mid-transverse colon and hepatic flexure.

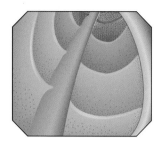

Fig 6.69 The longitudinal bulge of a tenia coli shows the axis of the colon.

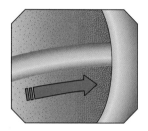

Fig 6.70 Follow the longitudinal bulge (tenia coli) round an acute bend.

The longitudinal fold of the ante-mesenteric tenia coli may bulge into a voluminous transverse colon, which is a useful pointer to the correct axis—rather like the white line down the center of a road (Fig 6.69). Appreciating this is particularly helpful at very acute angulations, as occurs when the mid-transverse colon is pushed down by the endoscope; a tenia coli can be followed blindly to push or angulate round the bend and see the lumen beyond (Fig 6.70).

After passing the mid-point of the transverse, it may be slow and difficult, with considerable push-pressure needed, to "climb the hill" up the proximal limb of the looped transverse colon (Fig 6.71a, Video 6.17). In some patients this aggressive approach can be avoided if the transverse colon can be shortened by deflating it and pulling back vigorously. The tip, being hooked around the transverse loop, then lifts up and flattens the transverse (Fig 6.71b) so that the tip advances as the shaft is withdrawn. This is the phenomenon of "paradoxical movement." Hand-pressure can be helpful, whether over the sigmoid colon during inward push or in the left hypochondrium to lift up the transverse loop. If there are problems, change of position (usually to left lateral position, sometimes to supine, right lateral, or even prone positions) can also help.

When the tip is established in the proximal transverse colon *counterclockwise torque* often helps it to advance toward the hepatic flexure. This useful phenomenon results from flattening out of the counterclockwise spiral formed by the shaft running anteriorly and medially around the splenic flexure from the descending colon to the transverse colon (Video 6.17).

In the transverse colon—to reach the hepatic flexure:
1 *pull back to lift up the transverse loop*
2 *deflate*
3 *try counterclockwise twist*
4 *try hand-pressure in the upper abdomen*
5 *. . . or hand-pressure over the sigmoid.*

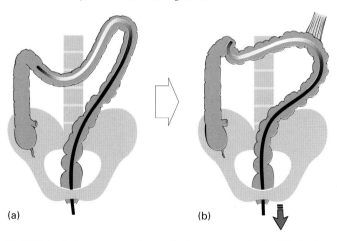

(a)   (b)

Fig 6.71 (a) If the passage up the proximal transverse colon is difficult, (b) pull back to lift and shorten it.

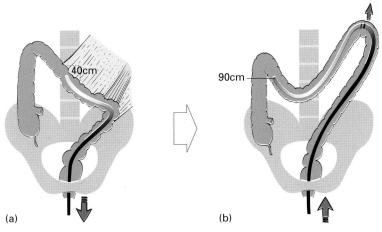

Fig 6.72 (a) If the phrenicocolic ligament is lax, withdrawal maneuvers are ineffective, (b) and pushing in simply re-forms the loop.

A mobile splenic flexure may adversely affect "transverse lift" maneuvers. The fulcrum or cantilever effect caused by the phrenicocolic ligament fixing the normal splenic flexure is crucial. In some patients this attachment is lax, allowing the splenic flexure to be pulled back to 40 cm (rather than the usual 50 cm rule) (Fig 6.72a); the colon is then found to be hypermobile and unresponsive to any of the normally effective withdrawal or twisting movements (Fig 6.72b). When this occurs the use of force is ineffectual, but deflation, counterclockwise twist, hand-pressure, posturing (usually in left lateral but sometimes to right lateral), and gentle perseverance will coax the tip up to the hepatic flexure. Simple aggression and force usually worsens the loop, whereas subtlety and patience often win.

A gamma loop may form in a very long redundant transverse colon (Fig 6.73), as can be well seen using the magnetic imager (Video 6.18). A gamma loop is large and rarely removable, both because of its sheer size (conflicting with the small intestine and other organs during attempted de-rotation) and because colon mobility makes it difficult to find any point where angulation will anchor the tip. The instrument therefore falls back each time it is withdrawn and it is necessary to to push on to the cecum with the loop in place.

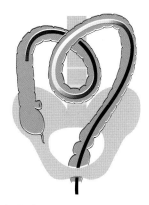

Fig 6.73 A gamma loop in a redundant transverse colon.

On the rare occasions that a gamma loop is successfully removed, this is by combined withdrawal and very strong twist (usually counterclockwise) to lift up the transverse colon into a more conventional position. Having the magnetic imager available greatly increases the chance of success, because it shows very obviously which twist to apply, and whether the de-rotation maneuver is starting to work. Using the magnetic imager it is also sometimes possible to prevent a gamma loop, twisting strongly counterclockwise and pulling back to keep the transverse shorter.

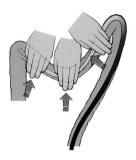

Fig 6.74 "Specific" hand-pressure may elevate the transverse colon.

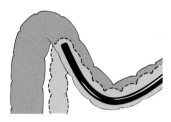

Fig 6.75 Aspirate to shrink the hepatic flexure toward the scope.

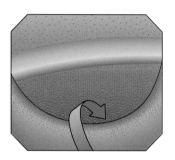

Fig 6.76 Suction toward, then angle acutely (180°) around the acute hepatic flexure.

Hand-pressure over the transverse or sigmoid colon

Hand-pressure is helpful in about 30% of transverse colons, reducing the tendency for scope looping within the abdominal cavity and encouraging as straight a line as possible to the hepatic flexure and cecum. The rationale for pressure in the lower left abdomen over the looping sigmoid colon has been described (see Fig 6.60), and the tendency of the sigmoid to re-loop at all stages of the examination has also been mentioned. Because of this tendency, hand-pressure over the sigmoid colon is a good bet whenever the instrument is looping (even in the transverse), and its application has therefore been called *"nonspecific" hand-pressure*.

Brief and gentle initial hand-pressure may affect the transverse colon, providing that it passes close enough to the abdominal wall to be accessible. This maneuver has been called *"specific" hand-pressure*. In the proximal colon, at any time that a few extra centimeters of insertion are needed but cannot be achieved, try abdominal hand-pressure—first "nonspecific" (in the left lower abdomen) but, if this fails use "specific" pressure, according to the results of local palpation, in either:
- *the left hypochondrium region* (to push the whole loop toward the hepatic flexure)
- *the mid-abdomen* (to counteract the sagging transverse colon) (Fig 6.74)
- *the right hypochondrium* (to impact directly on the hepatic flexure).

Hepatic flexure

The hepatic flexure (Video 6.19) is, from both an anatomical and endoscopic viewpoint, a nearly 180° hairpin bend, similar in many respects to the bend at the sigmoid–descending junction but more constant in its fixation and more voluminous.

Passing the hepatic flexure

1 *Assess from a distance* the correct direction around the flexure because, after the tip reaches into it, it is so close to the opposing mucosa that it is very difficult to steer except by a predetermined plan. At all costs avoid impacting the tip forcibly against the opposing wall or it will catch in the haustral folds and there will be no view at all.
2 *Aspirate air carefully* from the hepatic flexure, to collapse it toward, but not actually onto, the tip as it moves around (Fig 6.75).
3 *Ask the patient to breathe in* (and hold the breath), which lowers the diaphragm, and often the flexure too.
4 *Steer the tip blindly in the previously determined direction* around the flexure. As the hepatic flexure is very acute, it takes some confidence to angulate nearly 180° around in the same direction without seeing well (Fig 6.76). Use both angulation controls simultaneously to achieve full angulation; adding clockwise twist may be helpful.

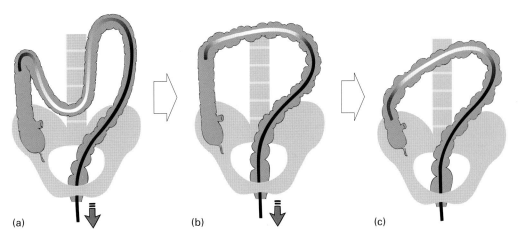

Fig 6.77 (a) When around the hepatic flexure and viewing the ascending colon, (b) pull back to straighten, (c) and aspirate to collapse the colon and pass toward the cecum.

5 *Withdraw the instrument* substantially for up to 30–50 cm to lift up the transverse colon and straighten out the colonoscope (Fig 6.77a,b) for passage into the ascending colon.

6 *Try upper abdominal hand-pressure.*

7 *Aspirate air again* once the ascending colon is seen, in order to shorten the colon and drop the colonoscope down toward the cecum (Fig 6.77c).

A combination of these maneuvers is used simultaneously. Aspiration brings the hepatic flexure toward the tip until the inner fold of the flexure can be passed, the colonoscope is withdrawn (either by manipulation of the shaft or by the endoscopist pulling the colonoscope out, using both hands simultaneously to work the angulation controls), and the tip is steered maximally around until it can be sucked down into the ascending colon. A parallel has already been drawn between the "hook, withdraw, and clockwise twist" situation in the transverse loop and hepatic flexure and the "right twist and withdrawal" method of shortening the sigmoid N-loop at the sigmoid–descending colon angle. The same instrument maneuvers apply to both, except that they must be exaggerated at the hepatic flexure because of its larger dimensions.

Position change

Position change is another trick that helps coax the colonoscope tip into and around the hepatic flexure. Change the patient's position (to supine, prone, or sometimes even right lateral position) if there is difficulty in passing in the usual left lateral position. Using brute force at the hepatic flexure rarely pays off, since the combined sigmoid and transverse colon loops can take up most of the length of even a long colonoscope shaft. With the instrument really straightened at the hepatic flexure, only about 70 cm of the shaft should remain in the patient (this is one of the situations where a distance check helps to ensure that the colonoscope is straight and results in easy and painless insertion).

Is it the hepatic flexure—or might it be the splenic?

A final, embarrassing, point is that if things are not working out at the hepatic flexure after applying the various tips, the colonoscope may actually still be at the splenic flexure. In a redundant colon it is possible to be overoptimistic and get hopelessly lost. The clue to this is often that the hepatic flexure (in left lateral position) is dry or air-filled, whereas the splenic is likely to be fluid-filled.

Ascending colon and ileo-cecal region

Endoscopic anatomy

The ascending colon is posteriorly placed at its origin from the hepatic flexure, but then runs anteriorly so that where it joins the cecum it is just under the anterior abdominal wall and usually accessible to finger palpation or transillumination. In 90% of subjects, the ascending colon and cecum are predictably fixed retroperitoneally, but the remainder may be mobile on a persistent mesocolon, with correspondingly variable positions.

The cecum is an evolutionarily defunct and stagnant part of the colon proximally, between the point of entry of the ileo-cecal valve and the appendix orifice. It is typically about 5 cm in length, but sometimes surprisingly capacious and difficult to examine properly. Being out of the normal stream, the cecum is often poorly prepared and may require irrigation for proper views. The *cecal sling fold*, well known to surgeons, typically results in anterior angulation of the cecum. This angulation is why the cecum and appendix may be poorly seen from the ascending colon and why position change (to partially prone or supine) can help the scope slide toward the cecal pole and appendix.

At the pole of the cecum the three teniae coli may fuse around the appendix (crow's-foot or "Mercedes Benz sign") (Fig 6.78), but the anatomy is somewhat variable. Between the teniae coli and the marked cecal haustra there can be cavernous outpouchings, which are difficult to examine.

The appendix orifice is normally an unimpressive slit, which is often crescentic because the appendix is folded around the cecum. Because the appendix is characteristically flexed toward the center of the abdomen, it can give guidance as to the likely site of entry of the ileum (see "Finding the ileo-cecal valve," below). Only rarely is the appendix orifice seen straight-on as a tube, probably when the cecum is fully mobile. The appendix may sometimes be less than obvious at the center of a local whirl of mucosal folds—not unlike a Danish pastry. The operated appendix usually looks no different unless it has been eradicated entirely or invaginated into a stump, when it can sometimes resemble a polyp (take care—perhaps take a biopsy but do not attempt polypectomy!).

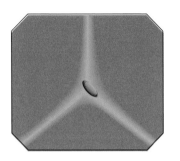

Fig 6.78 Appendix orifice at the fusion of the three teniae coli.

The ileo-cecal valve (Video 6.20) is on the prominent ileo-cecal fold encircling the cecum about 5 cm back from its pole. Unfortunately for the endoscopist, the orifice of the valve is often a slit on the invisible upstream or "cecal" aspect of the ileo-cecal fold. The most the endoscopist normally sees is the slight bulge of the upper lip. It is therefore rare to see the orifice directly without specific close-up maneuvers.

Reaching the cecum

On seeing the ascending colon the temptation is to push in, but this usually results in the transverse loop re-forming and the tip sliding back. The secret is to deflate. The resulting collapse of the capacious hepatic flexure and ascending colon will drop the tip downward toward the cecum (see Fig 6.77c); it also lowers the position of the hepatic flexure relative to the splenic flexure and, with this mechanical advantage, pushing inward should become more effective. Aspirate and steer carefully down the center of the deflating lumen, then push the last few centimeters into the cecum. If it proves difficult to reach the last few centimeters to the cecal pole, change the patient's position to semi-prone (even a partial position change of 20–30° may help) or, if that does not work, change to supine position. Once in the cecum, the bowel can be reinflated to get a better view.

The cecum can be voluminous with pronounced haustral infoldings and tendency to spasm, making it confusing to examine. In particular, it is possible to be mistaken about whether the pole has actually been reached. One catch is that the ileo-cecal valve fold, the major circumferential fold at the junction of the ascending colon and the cecum—on which is situated the give-away bulge of the valve—has a tendency to be in tonic spasm. The contracted fold may easily be mistaken by the unwary either for the appendix orifice or for the ileo-cecal valve. Insufflating and pushing in with the instrument tip and/or using *extra IV antispasmodic* medication will reveal the cavernous cecal pole beyond.

Be careful to identify landmarks before assuming "total colonoscopy" has been performed. The appendix orifice and ileo-cecal valve should be identified as positive landmarks. "Soft" but suggestive evidence is given by seeing right iliac fossa transillumination (Fig 6.79) or finger-palpation indenting the cecal region (Fig 6.80). At the same time the colonoscope should, after withdrawal, be at 70–80 cm. The cecal pole is often difficult to examine, not always completely clean and sometimes in tonic spasm; a "too good to be true" appearance may therefore actually be only the ascending colon (or even the hepatic flexure). Inability to locate the ileo-cecal valve opening and noting that the shaft distance on withdrawal is only at 60–70 cm should warn of this possibility.

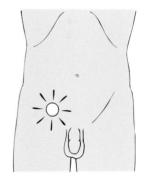

Fig 6.79 Transillumination deep in the iliac fossa suggests the cecum.

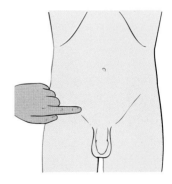

Fig 6.80 Finger-pressure in the right iliac fossa indents the cecum.

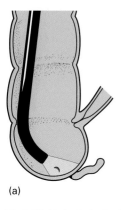

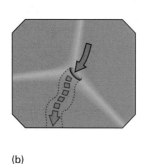

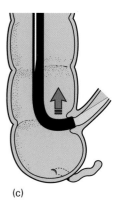

(a)   (b)   (c)

Fig 6.81 (a) Angle in the direction of the appendix lumen, (b) and pull back until the proximal lip of the ileo-cecal valve rides up into the view.

Finding the ileo-cecal valve

The "appendix trick" or "bow and arrow" sign (Video 6.20) is an ingenious way of finding the ileo-cecal valve, and simultaneously entering the ileum too—a "double whammy" when it works first time.

1 *Find the appendix orifice* (Fig 6.81a).

2 *Imagine an arrow* pointing in the direction of the appendix lumen (Fig 6.81b).

3 *Angulate in that direction and pull back* (still angled) for about 3–4 cm (Fig 6.81c).

4 At this point expect the proximal lip of the ileo-cecal valve to start to ride up over the lens, with shiny bumps of close-up ileal villi apparent, rather than the mirror-smooth crypt-spotted colon mucosa.

5 Slowly insufflate and twist or angulate gently to wangle into the ileum.

The "appendix trick" succeeds when (as is usual) the appendix is bent toward the center of the abdomen, from which direction the ileum also enters the cecum. The appendix effectively acts as an indicator of direction (rather as an airport windsock indicates wind direction).

The other way to find the valve is to pull back about 8–10 cm from the cecal pole and to look for the first prominent circular haustral fold, around 5 cm back from the pole. On this "ileo-cecal" fold will be the telltale thickening or bulge of the ileo-cecal valve. A common mistake is to look for the valve when the endoscope tip is in the cecal pole, rather than pulling back to the mid-ascending colon to get a proper overall view from a distance. Looking at this ileo-cecal fold, with the cecum moderately inflated, one part of it should be seen to be less perfectly concave than the rest. It may be simply flattened out, bulge in (especially on deflation when it often bulges more obviously and may bubble or issue ileal contents), show a characteristic "buttock-like" double bulge, or, less commonly, have obvious protuberant lips or a "volcano" appearance (Fig 6.82). It is rather uncommon to see the actual slit orifice or pouting lips of the valve straight on, because the opening is nor-

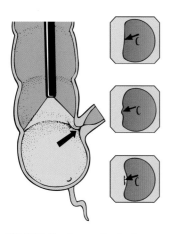

Fig 6.82 The ileo-cecal valve is a bulge on the ileo-cecal fold—a flattening, single, or double bulge or a "volcano."

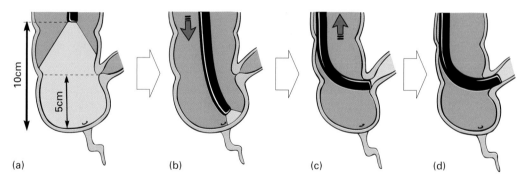

Fig 6.83 (a) Locate the ileo-cecal valve, (b) insert beyond, angulate, and deflate slightly, (c) pull back until the "red out" is seen, (d) and insufflate to open the valve.

mally on the cecal side of the ileo-cecal fold. The best the endo-scopist can usually achieve is a partial, close-up, and tangential view, and often only after careful maneuvering. Change of patient position may be helpful if the initial view is poor or disadvantageous for tip entry.

Entering the ileum

"Direct entry" into the ileum is made easier by a combination of actions.

1 *Rehearse at a distance* (about 10 cm back from the cecal pole) the easiest steering movements, preferably combining shaft twist and down-angulation to point the tip toward the valve (Fig 6.83a). If possible rotate the endoscope so that the valve lies in the downward (6 o'clock) position relative to the tip, because this allows entry with an easy downward angulation movement (lateral or oblique movements are more awkward single-handedly) and because the tip air outlet is situated below the lens, but needs to enter the valve first in order to open up the ileum with insufflation.

2 *Pass the colonoscope tip* in over the ileo-cecal valve fold in the region of the valvular bulge and angle in toward the valve (Fig 6.83b). Overshoot a little, so that the action of angulation directs the tip into the opening, not short of it.

3 *Deflate the cecum partially* to make the valve supple (Fig 6.83b).

4 *Pull back the scope*, angling downward until the tip catches in the soft lips of the valve, resulting in a "red out" of transilluminated tissue (Fig 6.83c), typically with the telltale granular appearance of the villous surface in close-up (as opposed to the pale shine of colonic mucosa).

5 *On seeing the "red out," freeze all movement.*

6 Then *insufflate air* to open the lips (Fig 6.83d) and wait, gently twisting or angling the scope a few millimeters if necessary until the direction of the ileal lumen becomes apparent. If considerable angulation has been used to enter the valve, *de-angulation* may be needed to straighten things out and let the tip slide in.

7 *Multiple attempts may be needed for success*, both in locating the valve and entering the ileum, if necessary rotating to slightly different parts of the ileo-cecal fold, hooking over it and pulling back

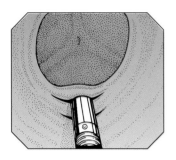

Fig 6.84 The biopsy forceps can be used to locate the slit of the valve, and then pass into it.

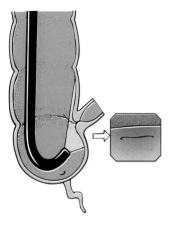

Fig 6.85 A slit-like valve may only be visible in retroversion (in a large colon).

to pass the area repeatedly. On each successive attempt try to learn from the problems of the previous one, fining down tip movements to a centimeter or two and a few degrees either way. Change of patient position may also help.

8 *The biopsy forceps can be used as a guidewire*. If only a distant, partial, or uncertain view can be obtained of the ileal bulge or opening, it is possible to use the biopsy forceps to locate and then pass into the opening of the valve (Fig 6.84), either to obtain a blind biopsy or to act as an "anchor." The forceps fix the position of the tip relative to the valve and facilitate endoscope passage through it (as with a guidewire). Even if entry into the ileum is not intended, the opened forceps can be used to hook back the bulge of the upper lip of the valve to visualize the ileal opening and make identification certain.

Entry into the ileum can be in retroflexion. This "last-ditch" maneuver is only likely to work in a huge colon and if the scope is completely straightened and responsive. It is a useful option when the ileo-cecal valve is slit-like and invisible from above (Fig 6.85). Retrovert the tip to visualize and then to enter the valve from below (Fig 6.86a). Very acute angulation of the colonoscope tip is needed, with maximum up/down and lateral angulation, and often some twist of the shaft as well. Fairly forceful inward push may be needed to impact low enough in the cecal pole to visualize the valve. The extra length of the bending section of video endoscopes, due to the CCD electronics, means that in a normal-sized colon the tip retroverts into mid-ascending with no view of the valve. In those few cases that the valve can be seen, pull back to impact the tip within it (Fig 6.86b), insufflate to open the lips and de-angulate and pull back further to enter the ileum, with or without use of the forceps (Fig 6.86c).

Problems in entering the ileo-cecal valve occur for a number of reasons. The endoscope may be in the hepatic flexure, not the cecum. Even if the tip is in the right place, the chosen "bulge" on the ileo-cecal valve fold may not be correct; some valve openings are entirely flat and slit-like (Fig 6.87a), effectively invisible on the reverse side of the fold. It is a mistake to aim the objective lens (at the center of the endoscope tip) exactly at the slit, which may result

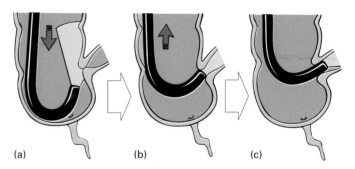

(a)   (b)   (c)

Fig 6.86 (a) If necessary retroflex to see the valve, (b) pull back to impact, (c) and insufflate and de-angulate to enter the ileum.

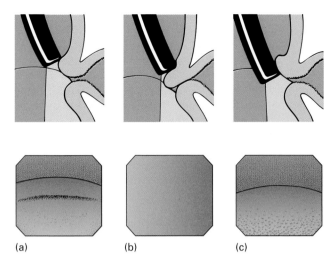

(a)   (b)   (c)

Fig 6.87 Entering the ileo-cecal valve. (a) Distant view of the valve slit. (b) Pushing in directly may impact against the upper lip. (c) Overshooting the valve lets the tip angulate in successfully.

in impaction of the scope tip against the upper lip of the valve (Fig 6.87b). This is why overshooting the opening slightly (Fig 6.87c) will let the angled tip edge in to the ileum successfully, even though the initial view has been less good.

Those cases of active inflammatory disease (especially Crohn's) where the colonoscopist wants to see the terminal ileum are also those where the valve is most likely to be narrowed and, although a limited view may be possible and biopsies taken, the valve may be impassable. Conversely in some cases of longstanding, chronic, or healed previous colitis the valve may be atrophic and widely patent, without the usual soft or bulging lips.

Inspecting the terminal ileum

The terminal ileum surface looks granular in air, but underwater the villi float up prettily—like coral or lambs' wool. The ileal surface is often studded with raised lymphoid follicles resembling small polyps, or these can be aggregated into plaque-like Peyer's patches. Sometimes the ileum is surprisingly colon-like, with a pale shiny surface and visible submucosal vascular pattern. After colon resection the difference between colon and ileum may be imperceptible because of villus atrophy. Using dye spray (0.1% indigo carmine) to highlight the surface detail will rapidly discriminate between the granular or "sandpaper" appearance of the ileal mucosa and the small circumferential grooves of the colonic surface, which give a "fingerprint" effect.

The ileum is soft, peristaltic, and collapsible compared with the colon. Rather than attempting forceful insertion, greater distances can be traversed by gentle steering and deflation, so that the intestine collapses over the colonoscope. At each acute bend it is best to deflate a little, hook round, pull back, and then steer gently (if necessary almost blindly) around and inward before pulling back again to relocate the direction of view—a "two steps forward and one step back" approach that applies throughout colonoscopy. When the colonoscope tip is in the ileum, it can often be passed in up to 30–50 cm with care and patience, although this length of intestine may be folded on to only about 20 cm of instrument. Air distension in the small intestine should be kept to a minimum because it is particularly uncomfortable and slow to clear after examination—another reason for routinely using CO_2.

Examination of the colon

The aim of colonoscopy is to see all parts of the colon as well as possible. The images that can be obtained with modern high-definition colonoscopes are impressive, but the endoscopist may have to work hard to achieve them. The most obvious problems of colonoscopy occur during insertion, which is why so much text has been devoted to overcoming them. However, the 6–8 minutes that should be taken to examine on withdrawal are the most critical. During this withdrawal phase the endoscopist must be dexterous, but also slow and obsessional in trying to minimize blind spots—suctioning puddles, irrigating any residue, and being prepared to reinsert and reexamine each fold or loop that may have been inadequately viewed. Examination (video 6.21) should involve just as much skill and hard work as insertion, with intense visual concentration so as to maximize the yield of even small or flat adenomas among the folds of the colon.

Better views are obtained during withdrawal than on insertion, so more painstaking examination is usually performed on the way out. However, in many areas, especially around bends, a different and sometimes much better view is obtained during insertion. For this reason, when a perfect view is obtained of a small polyp or other lesion during insertion it is better to deal with it at once (snare, biopsy, or image, as appropriate) rather than have the humbling experience of not being able to find it again on the way out and thereby waste time. A convincing example to the endoscopist who doubts this difference between insertion and withdrawal is in the larger number of diverticular orifices seen while inserting around bends (so the colon wall is seen side-on) compared with the relatively few seen on formal examination on the way out.

The colon is shortened and crumpled during insertion and, during withdrawal, the most convoluted or crumpled parts (such as the transverse and sigmoid colon) can spring off the tip at such speed that it is difficult to ensure a complete view. At sharp bends or marked haustrations there may therefore be blind spots during a single withdrawal. Careful scanning and twisting movements should be used in an attempt to survey all parts of each haustral fold or bend, and some may need to be reexamined several times. At a flexure the outside of the bend may be seen on the first pass, but the colonoscope often has to be reinserted and hooked to get a selective view of the other side. Acute bends, including the hepatic and splenic flexures, the sigmoid–descending colon junction, and the capacious parts of the cecum and rectum, are potential blind spots where the endoscopist needs to take particular care to avoid "misses" (Fig 6.88).

Changes of position can help proper inspection. The splenic flexure and descending colon are rapidly filled with air and emptied of fluid by asking the patient to rotate toward the right lateral position. It is our policy routinely to rotate patients briefly to the right oblique position for inspection of the left colon (splenic flexure and descending colon), then back to the left lateral position again for a better view of the sigmoid colon and rectum.

Single-handed technique comes into its own during inspection on withdrawal. The endoscopist has precise control and the corkscrewing movements made by twisting the shaft are the quickest way of scanning a bend or haustral fold so that a problem area can rapidly be reexamined several times. Using an assistant for two-person handling creates difficulties of communication and coordination that make it much more difficult to be thorough and accurate.

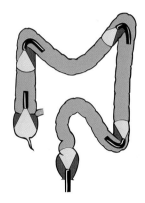

Fig 6.88 Potential blind spots for colonoscopic visualization.

As well as being obsessional, the endoscopist must be honest, reporting not only what is seen but also when the view has been imperfect due to technical difficulty or bad bowel preparation. Even during an ideal examination, the endoscopist probably misses at least 5–10% of the mucosal surface, and in a problematic examination may miss up to 20–30% (although large protuberant lesions are less likely to be missed). Anyone who doubts this should read both the "tandem colonoscopy" or "back to back studies," in which two skilled colonoscopists examine the same patient on the same visit, and the comparisons with CT colography, reporting a 12–17% "miss" rate of large (1 cm) adenomas by colonoscopy. Similarly reported "adenoma-detection rates" vary enormously between scrupulous, careful, slower endoscopists and the "speed merchants," who should not be involved in screening and surveillance programs.

Quality control of colonoscopy is a difficult matter, but endoscopists can (and should) be assessed on their validated cecal completion rate, adenoma detection rate during screening exams, and the time taken for withdrawal. Continuous quality improvement (CQI) programs now form part of many societies' recommendations on credentialing and monitoring for colonoscopy. As part of this there are obvious possibilities for advanced simulation to provide objective testing of dexterity and accuracy in polyp detection in a range of standardized, simulated, colons.

Localization

Uncertainty in localization is one of the endoscopist's most serious problems, especially during flexible sigmoidoscopy or limited colonoscopy, but even during supposed "total" or complete colonoscopy. This can lead to mistakes in judging where the instrument has reached and therefore which maneuvers to employ. Endoscopic errors of localization can also be catastrophic if the surgeon is given wrong information around which to plan a resection.

Distance of insertion of the instrument is inaccurate. Although sometimes used by inexperienced colonoscopists to express the

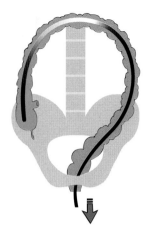

Fig 6.89 Pulling back the scope shortens the colon.

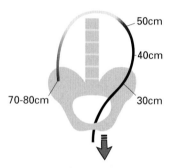

Fig 6.90 If the scope is in the cecum at 70–80 cm, other anatomical sites are predictable by measurement.

position of the instrument or of lesions found ("the colonoscope was inserted to 90 cm," "a polyp was seen at 30 cm," etc.). Distance of insertion does not give an accurate measurement. The elasticity of the colon makes such information meaningless; at 70 cm the instrument may be in the sigmoid colon, in the cecum, or anywhere between. On withdrawal, however, assuming a fully straightened scope, providing no adhesions are present and mesenteric fixations are normal, the colon will shorten and straighten predictably (Fig 6.89) so that measurement gives approximate localization. On withdrawal, the cecum should be at 70–80 cm, the transverse colon at 60 cm, the splenic flexure at 50 cm, the descending colon at 40 cm, and the sigmoid colon at 30 cm (Fig 6.90). The last two values depend, of course, on the sigmoid colon being straightened. It is sometimes difficult to convince enthusiasts for rigid procto-sigmoidoscopy that at 25 cm their instrument may still be in the rectum, whereas the flexible colonoscope (on withdrawal) may be in the proximal sigmoid colon. Equally, it is sometimes possible for the colonoscope to be withdrawn to 55–60 cm when the tip is in the cecum.

Anatomical localization during insertion is inaccurate. In almost half the cases of a personal series the expert was wrong! In 25%, a persistent loop (spiral or "N") caused the endoscopist to judge the tip location to be at the splenic flexure when actually it was at the sigmoid–descending colon junction. In 20%, a mobile splenic flexure pulled down to 40 cm from the anus, causing the endoscopist wrongly to judge the instrument to be at the sigmoid––descending colon junction (see Fig 6.57). Similar inaccuracies are demonstrated by magnetic imager series.

The internal appearances of the colon can be misleading. In the sigmoid and descending colon the haustra and the colonic outline are generally circular (see Fig 6.11), whereas the longitudinal muscle straps or teniae coli cause the characteristic triangular cross section often seen in the transverse colon (see Fig 6.59). The descending colon, however, may look triangular or the transverse colon circular in outline. Visible evidence of extracolonic viscera normally occurs at the hepatic flexure, where there is seen to be a bluish/gray contact with the liver, but similar contact with external structures can occur at the splenic flexure or descending colon. The combination of an acute bend with sharp haustra and blue coloration is characteristic of the hepatic flexure and is a useful, but not infallible, endoscopic landmark. Pulsation of adjacent arteries is seen in the sigmoid colon (left common iliac artery), transverse colon (aorta), and sometimes in the ascending colon (right iliac).

The ileo-cecal valve is the only definite anatomical landmark in the colon, with villi often visible, but it has been stressed already that it is not always easy to find, and mistaken identification is possible unless the ileum is entered or the orifice and villi visualized.

Fluid levels can be surprisingly useful clues to localization, especially after oral lavage. Historically radiological routine was to rotate the patient into the right lateral or left lateral position to fill the dependent parts of the colon with barium (Fig 6.91). The endoscopist (with the patient in the usual left lateral position)

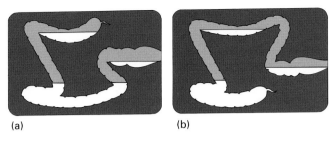

(a)   (b)

Fig 6.91 Barium enema in (a) the left lateral position and (b) the right lateral position.

knows that the instrument tip is in the descending colon when it enters fluid (see Fig 6.55), and is in the transverse colon when it leaves the fluid for the triangular and air-filled lumen of the transverse colon. However, a long transverse colon, when it sags down, can also contain a large amount of fluid, so mobile colons are particularly difficult for localization (and everything else).

Transillumination of the abdominal wall can be helpful if other imaging modalities are not available, but in obese patients this may necessitate a completely dark room. It should be remembered that the descending colon is so far posterior that no light is usually visible and that the surface marking of the splenic and hepatic flexures is by transillumination through the rib cage posteriorly. Light in the right iliac fossa is suggestive, but not conclusive, that the instrument is in the cecum; similar appearances can be produced if the tip stretches and transilluminates the sigmoid or mid-transverse colon.

Finger indentation, palpation, or balloting can be effective, particularly in the ascending colon or cecum, where close apposition to the abdominal wall should make the impression of a palpating finger easily visible to the endoscopist, unless the patient is obese. If in doubt indent in several places and beware the possibility of transmitted forces giving misleading impressions, literally.

Location of the instrument tip or of lesions found during colonoscopy should therefore be made by the endoscopist in broad anatomical terms (e.g. "the polyp was seen on withdrawing the instrument at 30 cm in the proximal sigmoid colon"). The distance of instrument insertion may often be omitted altogether so that there is no chance of confusion in the mind of someone unfamiliar with the degree of shortening possible in the colon. Inaccurate localization can occur even when imaging is employed, and the endoscopist usually needs to rely on a combination of assessments—distance inserted, distance after withdrawal, and straightening of the shaft, endoscopic (and magnetic imager when available) appearances, and possibly visualization of palpating fingers or transillumination. Knowing the pitfalls and being careful should make localization reasonably accurate, but even experienced endoscopists can mistake the sigmoid colon for the splenic flexure, or the splenic flexure for the hepatic flexure, which can be a serious error if localizing a lesion before surgery.

Normal appearances

The colonic mucosa normally shows a generalized fine, ramifying vascular pattern, which can often be seen to be composed of parallel pairs of vessels comprising a venule (larger, bluer) and an arteriole (Video 6.22). The veins become particularly prominent in the rectum, notably so in the anal canal if a proctoscope is used to impede venous return and distend the hemorrhoidal plexus. The vessel pattern in the colon depends on the transparency of the normal colonic epithelium, as the vessels seen are in the submucosa. If the epithelial capillaries are dilated (as may occur after bowel preparation) the vascular pattern may be partly obscured. If hyperemia is marked (as in inflammatory bowel disease) there is no visible pattern. If the epithelial layer is thickened (as in the "atrophy" of inactive chronic inflammatory disease) the mucosa appears pale and featureless, even though biopsies may be essentially normal. The most convincing demonstration of how poorly the endoscopist normally sees the epithelial surface is to spray dye (0.1–0.4% indigo carmine) onto the colonic mucosa. Small irregularities and lymphoid follicles stand out and there is a fine interconnecting pattern of circumferential "innominate grooves" on the surface into which the dye sinks, providing there is no excess of mucus on the surface.

Prominent vessels should not be thought of as abnormal, and are not likely to be hemangiomatous or variceal unless they are markedly tortuous or serpentine. Mucosal trauma can occur during insertion of the colonoscope, and red or bloodstained patches may sometimes be seen on withdrawal, especially in the sigmoid or where the scope tip or looped sigmoid colon has traumatized other parts of the colon. Sometimes it may be wise to irrigate or to take biopsies to ensure that these appearances are not evidence of inflammatory change.

Abnormal appearances

It is not the purpose of this book to cover more than the most obvious points of endoscopic pathology, which are fully featured in the various available atlases of endoscopy (Video 6.23). Fortu- nately for the endoscopist, nearly all colonic abnormalities are either mucosal, with characteristic discoloration, or project into the lumen so that they are easy to see and excise or biopsy (Video 6.24).

Submucosal lesions

Submucosal lesions, which may be very difficult to diagnose, include secondary carcinoma, endometriosis, and a few large-vessel hemangiomas. The endoscopist has a poor appreciation of colonic contour as a result of distortion from the wide-angle lens and flat illumination of endoscopes. He or she may also see nothing, or remarkably little compared with the radiologist, of extracolonic communications such as tracks or fistulae. Any experienced endoscopist has, through bitter experience, learned humility in visual interpretation and also takes care to provide appropriate specimens for pathological opinion when relevant.

Polyps

The normal colonic mucosa is pale, so submucosal abnormalities are too, including lipomas or gas cysts. The *smallest polyps* (of whatever histology) are also pale and those of 1–2 mm diameter may be transparent and invisible except on light reflex or dye spray. In polyps 3–4 mm in diameter, there may equally be little difference in appearance between a normal mucosal excrescence and a hyperplastic, adenomatous or any other type of polyp, although small adenomas are more often red and frequently have a matt-looking or even brain-like ("gyral" or "sulcal") surface in close-up view. The combination of high-resolution or zoom endoscopes with vital staining (methylene blue) or surface enhancement by dye spraying (indigo carmine) or by narrow band imaging is able to give the endoscopist truly microscopic views, but the clinical impact that this will have is uncertain.

Narrow band imaging (NBI) is a technology that uses filtered bluish light to give enhanced views of the mucosal surface, provides exquisite detail of the vascularity of polyps and early cancers. Adenomas (compared with metaplastic polyps) are more vascular and appear dark brown in the field of view, a simple color change that aids detection.

Melanosis makes the smallest polyps easy to pick out if the patient has been a purgative taker, as the dusky appearance of melanosis coli (often most marked in the right colon) does not stain polyps, which stand out like pale islands, or the ileo-cecal valve.

Villous adenomas may be pale, soft and shiny, but have a rough surface; they are commonest in the rectum.

Larger hyperplastic or serrated polyps (7–15 mm in diameter and sessile) can occur in the proximal colon, when they typically appear brown and gelatinous because their surface mucus adsorbs bile. Viewed with NBI illumination they appear as pale as the surrounding normal mucosa.

Malignant polyps may be obviously irregular, may bleed easily from surface ulceration or be paler, and typically also firmer to palpation with the biopsy forceps. Such signs of possible malignancy in a stalked polyp warn the endoscopist to electrocoagulate the base thoroughly, to obtain a histological opinion on the stalk, and to localize and tattoo the polyp site carefully for follow-up and in case subsequent surgery is indicated.

Carcinomas

Carcinomas are usually very obvious. They are larger and have a more extensive and irregular base than a polyp. Ulcer cancers are uncommon in the colon but look like malignant gastric ulcers. However, small "early cancers" do occur, typically 6–20 mm in diameter with a slightly depressed center.

Conditions that can almost exactly mimic malignancy are granulation tissue masses at an anastomosis, larger granulation tissue polyps in chronic ulcerative colitis, and (rarely) the acute stage of an ischemic process. Biopsy evidence should always be obtained, bearing in mind that the pathologist may only be able to report "dysplastic tissue," as there may not be diagnostic evidence of invasive malignancy in the small pieces presented, which is why a snare-loop specimen should be taken whenever possible. Even with standard biopsy forceps, a surprisingly large specimen can be taken by the "avulsion" or "push biopsy" approach; the instrument is then withdrawn, keeping the forceps outside the tip so as not to shear off parts of the tissue by pulling it back through the biopsy channel.

Inflammatory bowel disease

Biopsies must always be taken in any patient with bowel frequency, loose stools, or any clinical suspicion of inflammatory disease (Videos 6.25 and 6.26). "Microscopic colitis," whether ulcerative or Crohn's, with clear abnormality on histology, can look absolutely normal to the endoscopist. Similarly "collagenous colitis," a rare cause of unexplained diarrhea due to an extensive "plate" of collagen under the epithelial surface, also appears normal endoscopically and the diagnosis can only be made on biopsies (at least four should be taken at intervals around the colon) in any patient with diarrhea.

Mucosal abnormality can vary enormously in different forms of inflammatory bowel disease. Inflamed mucosa can show the most minute haziness of vascular pattern, slight reddening, or a tendency to friability (easy bleeding). Colonoscopic biopsies rarely yield diagnostic granulomas in Crohn's disease, whereas the appearance of multiple, small, flat or volcano-like "aphthoid" ulcers set in a normal vascular pattern is characteristic. The differential diagnosis of the various specific and nonspecific inflammatory disorders may not be easy: infective conditions, ulcerative, ischemic, irradiation, and Crohn's colitis can all look amazingly similar in the acute stage, although biopsies will usually differentiate between them.

The ulcer from a previous rectal biopsy or a solitary ulcer of the rectum can look endoscopically identical to a Crohn's ulcer, whereas tuberculous ulcers are similar but more heaped up, and amebic ulcers more friable. Ulceration can also occur in chronic ulcerative colitis and ischemic disease but against a background of inflamed mucosa. The endoscopic appearances must be taken together with the clinical context and histological opinion. In the severe or chronic stage it is often impossible for either endoscopist or pathologist to be categoric in differential diagnosis.

Unexplained rectal bleeding, anemia, or occult blood loss

Blood loss or anemia is a common reason for undertaking colonoscopy. Although colonoscopy gives an impressive yield of radiologically missed cancers and polyps, 50–60% of patients will show no obvious abnormality, which raises the specter of whether anything has been missed.

Hemorrhoids can be seen with the colonoscope, often by retroversion in the rectum, but even better with a proctoscope used after colonoscope withdrawal. The colonoscope tip is inserted up the proctoscope (Fig 6.13) to show the patient the anorectal appearances or to take video-prints at "video-proctoscopy."

Hemangiomas are rare, but they can assume any appearance from massive and obvious submucosal discoloration with huge serpentine vessels to telangiectases or minute solitary nevi, which could easily be missed in folds or bends.

Angiodysplasias are uncommon and mainly occur in the cecum or ascending colon, but also in the small intestine. They have variable appearances, may be solitary or multiple (often two or three) and are always bright red, but they can be small vascular plaques, spidery telangiectases, or even a 1–2 mm dot lesion.

Stomas

If a finger can be inserted into any stoma, a standard or pediatric colonoscope will also pass without trouble, but a pediatric gastroscope can be substituted if necessary. It is quite normal for the stoma to change reactively to an unhealthy looking cyanotic color and even for there to be a little local bleeding, but no harm ensues.

Through an ileostomy, the distal 20 cm of ileum are easily examined (ideally with a pediatric colonoscope, enteroscope, or balloon endoscope), but further insertion depends on whether adhesions have formed. As in the sigmoid colon, the secret of passage through the small intestine is to pull the instrument back repeatedly as each bend is reached, which convolutes the intestine onto the instrument and straightens out the next short segment. Thus even though only 30–40 cm of instrument can be inserted, as much as 50–100 cm of intestine may be seen.

Colostomy patients are typically easy to examine, as the sigmoid colon will usually have been removed. The colon can be remarkably long, however, and full bowel preparation is essential. Colostomy washouts are less effective. The first few centimeters through the abdominal wall and proximal to the colostomy are sometimes awkward to negotiate and to examine, partly because of the continual escape of insufflated air. If there is a loop colostomy the afferent and efferent (proximal and distal) sides can be examined.

Pelvic ileo-anal pouches are easy to examine with a standard instrument. Limited examination of an ileal conduit is possible, using a pediatric endoscope (colonoscope or gastroscope).

Pediatric colonoscopy

Pediatric colonoscopy, from neonatal to 3–5 years of age, is best performed with a thinner (1 cm), preferably "floppy," pediatric colonoscope. In older children, depending on physique, adult colonoscopes can be used, and for teenagers they are mandatory. The infant anus will accept an adult little finger and so will take an endoscope of the same size. The neonatal sphincter first requires gentle dilation over a minute or two, using any small smooth tube (such as a nasogastric tube). The main advantage of a purpose-built pediatric colonoscope is more the extra flexibility or "softness" of its shaft than its small diameter. It is easy with stiffer adult colonoscopes to overstretch the mobile and elastic loops of a child's colon.

It is also generally a mistake to use a pediatric gastroscope because it is much stiffer.

Bowel preparation in children is usually very effective. Pleasant-tasting oral solutions such as senna syrup, magnesium citrate, or PEG–electrolyte are best tolerated. A saline enema will cleanse most of the colon of a baby, but phosphate enemas are contraindicated.

General anesthesia is frequently used, although children of any age can be colonoscoped without general anesthesia providing that the endoscopist is experienced. Reasonable IV medication is used, but a pediatrician with experience of resuscitation must be present as a safeguard. Neonates may sometimes be more safely examined with no sedation at all.

Per-operative colonoscopy

Exsanguinating bleeding is a rare indication for per-operative colonoscopy, because angiography is normally the preferred option. "On-table" cecostomy lavage preparation is used to give a reasonable view. Otherwise per-operative colonoscopy is normally only justified if attempts at colonoscopy have failed in a patient with known polyps, or where the colon proximal to a constricting neoplasm is to be inspected to exclude synchronous lesions at the time of resection.

Oral lavage or full colonoscopy bowel preparation must be used in nonobstructed patients, as most standard preoperative preparation regimens leave solid fecal residue. If the bowel has been completely obstructed, it is possible to perform on-table lavage through a temporary cecostomy tube or through a purse-string colotomy proximal to the obstructing lesion. During per-operative colonoscopy, overinsufflation of air can fill the small intestine and leave the surgeon with an unmanageable tangle of distended loops. This can be avoided if the endoscopist uses CO_2 insufflation instead of air, or if the surgeon places a clamp on the terminal ileum and the endoscopist aspirates carefully on withdrawal.

To examine the small intestine at laparotomy, in a Peutz–Jeghers patient for instance, if an enteroscope or balloon endoscope is not available a long (preferably variable stiffness) colonoscope can be used, either per-orally or through an intestinal incision; 70 cm of instrument is required to reach either the ligament of Treitz per-orally or the cecum per-anally. It helps if the surgeon either mobilizes or manually supports the fixed part of the duodenum (Fig 6.92) if the colonoscope is passed orally. The small intestine must be very gently handled on the endoscope to avoid local trauma or postoperative ileus. It is also important to insufflate as little as possible. Clamps are sequentially placed on each segment of small intestine after it has been evacuated. The surgeon inspects the transilluminated intestine from outside (with the room lights turned off) while the endoscopist inspects the inside. The surgeon marks any lesion to be resected with a stitch while the endoscopist can perform conventional snare polypectomies as appropriate. A

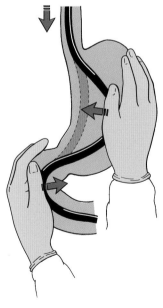

Fig 6.92 Per-operative straightening of the stomach and duodenum.

major source of confusion tends to be the artefactual submucosal hemorrhages that occur from handling the small intestine.

Further reading

General sources

Larsen WJ. *Human Embryology*. New York: Churchill Livingstone, 2001.

Waye JD, Rex DK, Williams CB. *Colonoscopy*. Oxford: Blackwell Publishing Ltd, 2009. *Extensively referenced multi-author textbook covering all aspects in detail—new edition in progress.*

Williams CB, Waye JD, Sakai Y. *Colonoscopy—the DVD*. Tokyo: Olympus Optical (& agents), 2003 or available from www.stmarkshospital.org.uk/shop/videos/colonoscopy-the-dvd.

Preparation, medication and management

Bell GD. Premedication, preparation, and surveillance. *Endoscopy* 2002; **34**: 2–12.

Bretthauer M, Lynge AB, Thiis-Evensen E, Hoff G, Fausa O, Aabakken L. Carbon dioxide insufflation in colonoscopy: safe and effective in sedated patients. *Endoscopy* 2005; **37**: 706–9.

Church J, Delaney C. Randomized, controlled trial of carbon dioxide insufflation during colonoscopy. *Dis Colon Rectum* 2003; **46**: 322–6.

East JE, Suzuki N, Arebi N, Bassett P, Saunders BP. Position changes improve visibility during colonoscope withdrawal: a randomized, blinded, crossover trial. *Gastrointest Endosc* 2007; **65**: 263–9.

Forbes GM, Collins BJ. Nitrous oxide for colonoscopy: a randomized controlled study. *Gastrointest Endosc* 2000; **51**: 271–7.

Froehlich F, Wietlisbach V, Gonvers JJ, Burnand B, Vader JP. Impact of colonic cleansing on quality and diagnostic yield of colonoscopy: the European Panel of Appropriateness of Gastrointestinal Endoscopy European multicenter study. *Gastrointest Endosc* 2005; **61**: 378–84.

Kim LS, Koch J, Yee J, Halvorsen R, Cello JP, Rockey DC. Comparison of patients' experiences during imaging tests of the colon. *Gastrointest Endosc* 2001; **54**: 67–74.

Martin JP, Sexton BF, Saunders BP, Atkin WS. Inhaled patient-administered nitrous oxide/oxygen mixture does not impair driving ability when used as analgesia during screening flexible sigmoidoscopy. *Gastrointest Endosc* 2000; **51**: 701–3.

Techniques and indications

Barclay RL, Vicari JJ, Doughty AS, Johanson JF, Greenlaw RL. Colonoscopic withdrawal times and adenoma detection during screening colonoscopy. *N Engl J Med* 2006; **355**: 2533–41.

Friedman S, Rubin PH, Bodian C, Goldstein E, Harpaz N, Present DH. Screening and surveillance colonoscopy in chronic Crohn's colitis. *Gastroenterology* 2001; **120**: 820–6.

Kiesslich R, Neurath MF. Surveillance colonoscopy in ulcerative colitis: magnifying chromoendoscopy in the spotlight. *Gut* 2004; **53**: 165–7.

Nelson DB. Technical assessment of direct colonoscopy screening: procedural success, safety, and feasibility. *Gastrointest Endosc Clin North Am* 2002; **12**: 77–84.

Rex DK. Colonoscopic withdrawal technique is associated with adenoma miss rates. *Gastrointest Endosc* 2000; **51**: 33–6.

Rex DK, Overley C, Kinser K *et al.* Safety of propofol administered by registered nurses with gastroenterologist supervision in 2000 endoscopic cases. *Am J Gastroenterol* 2002; **97**: 1159–63.

Saunders BP, Masaki T, Sawada T *et al*. A peroperative comparison of Western and Oriental colonic anatomy and mesenteric attachments. *Int J Colorectal Dis* 1995; **10**: 216–21.

Shah SG, Brooker JC, Williams CB, Thapar C, Suzuki N, Saunders BP. The variable stiffness colonoscope: assessment of efficacy by magnetic endoscope imaging. *Gastrointest Endosc* 2002; **56**: 195–201.

van Rijn JC, Reitsma JB, Stoker J, Bossuyt PM, van Deventer SJ, Dekker E. Polyp miss rate determined by tandem colonoscopy: a systematic review. *Am J Gastroenterol* 2006; **101**: 343–50.

Wexner SD, Garbus JE, Singh JJ. A prospective analysis of 13,580 colonoscopies. Reevaluation of credentialing guidelines. *Surg Endosc* 2002; **15**: 251–61.

Hazards and complications

Kavin RM, Sinicrope F, Esker AH. Management of perforation of the colon at colonoscopy. *Am J Gastroenterol* 1992; **87**: 161–7.

Rutgeerts P, Wang TH, Llorens PS, Zuccaro G, Jr. Gastrointestinal endoscopy and the patient with a risk of bleeding disorder. *Gastrointest Endosc* 1999; **49**: 134–6.

Tran DQ, Rosen L, Kim R, Riether RD, Stasik JJ, Khubchandani IT. Actual colonoscopy: what are the risks of perforation? *Am Surg* 2001; **67**: 845–7.

Chapter video clips

Video 6.1 History of colonoscopy
Video 6.2 Variable shaft stiffness
Video 6.3 ScopeGuide magnetic imager: The principles
Video 6.4 Embryology of the colon
Video 6.5 Insertion and handling of the colonoscope
Video 6.6 Steering the colonoscope
Video 6.7 Magnetic imager: An easy spiral loop
Video 6.8 Sigmoid loops
Video 6.9 Magnetic imager: Short and long "N"-loops
Video 6.10 Magnetic imager: "Alpha" spiral loops
Video 6.11 Magnetic imager: "Lateral view" spiral loop
Video 6.12 Magnetic imager: Flat "S"-loop in a long sigmoid
Video 6.13 Descending colon
Video 6.14 Splenic flexure
Video 6.15 Transverse colon
Video 6.16 Magnetic imager: Shortening transverse loops
Video 6.17 Magnetic imager: Deep transverse loops
Video 6.18 Magnetic imager: "Gamma" looping of the transverse colon
Video 6.19 Hepatic flexure
Video 6.20 Ileo-cecal valve
Video 6.21 Examination
Video 6.22 Normal appearances
Video 6.23 Abnormal appearances
Video 6.24 Post surgical appearances
Video 6.25 Infective colitis
Video 6.26 Crohn's Disease

Now check your understanding—go to
www.wiley.com/go/cottonwilliams/practicalgastroenterology

CHAPTER 7

Therapeutic Colonoscopy

Equipment

The equipment requirements for endoscopic polypectomy are few, and in many ways the fewer the better. It adds significantly to safety to be completely familiar with one electrosurgical unit, and only a few accessories, as from this familiarity it becomes easy to recognize when polypectomy is going right and when it is not.

Snare loops

Several makes of snare loop are available. Wire thickness and loop shape affect control of polypectomy. Single-use snares have the advantage of always being in good condition and predictable. Many endoscopists prefer to use a standard larger snare (2.5 cm diameter) and a "mini-snare" (9–10 mm diameter) for smaller polyps (Fig 7.1). The choice is mainly a matter of personal preference.

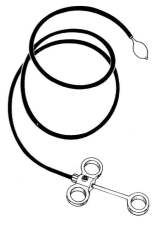

Fig 7.1 Use one commercial snare type for familiarity.

With any snare there are several points that should be checked *before* starting polypectomy:

1 *A smooth "feel" is essential for safety*. The snare handle and wire should open and close easily so that the endoscopist (or assistant) can estimate what is happening if the snare loop is out of view behind the polyp or its stalk. Single-use, disposable accessories avoid this, but if a reusable snare is being used and the inner wire has become bent and no longer moves freely it should be discarded.

2 *Snare wire thickness* greatly affects the speed of electrocoagulation and transection. Most loops are made of relatively thick wire so that there is little risk of cheese-wiring unintentionally and there is a larger contact area, which favors good local coagulation rather than electro-cutting. Some single-use snares have thin wire loops and need a lower current setting or extra care in closure to avoid cutting too rapidly, before full coagulation of stalk vessels. Be careful if using an unfamiliar snare type.

3 *Squeeze pressure* is very important, especially when snaring large polyps. There should be a 15 mm closure of the wire loop into the snare outer tube before use (Fig 7.2a). This ensures that the loop will squeeze the stalk tightly even if the plastic outer sheath crumples slightly under pressure, a particular problem with large stalks. If squeeze pressure is inadequate (Fig 7.2b) the final cut may have to rely entirely on using high-power electrical cutting and may not coagulate the central stalk vessels enough, with potentially disastrous (bleeding) consequences. If the loop closes too

Yes

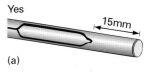

(a)

No

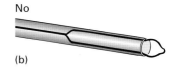

(b)

No

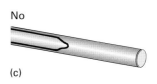

(c)

Fig 7.2 (a) Snare closed 15·mm is right; (b) wire too loose; (c) wire too tight.

Cotton and Williams' Practical Gastrointestinal Endoscopy: The Fundamentals, Seventh Edition.
Adam Haycock, Jonathan Cohen, Brian P Saunders, Peter B Cotton, and Christopher B Williams.
© 2014 John Wiley & Sons, Ltd. Published 2014 by John Wiley & Sons, Ltd.
Companion Website: www.wiley.com/go/cottonwilliams/practicalgastroenterology

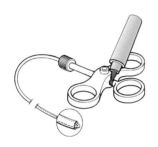

Fig 7.3 Mark the handle when the loop is fully closed.

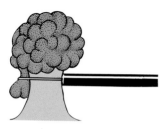

Fig 7.4 Polyp tissue can be trapped in the snare, reducing its efficiency.

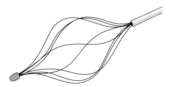

Fig 7.5 Multi-wire "memory metal" basket.

far (Fig 7.2c), cheese-wiring can occur before electrocoagulation is applied. This can also result in bleeding.

4 In addition, if the polyp is large, the view is poor or there is any reason to expect difficulty, ***mark the snare handle with a pencil or indelible pen*** at the point that the snare is just closed to the tip of the outer sheath (Fig 7.3). This is arguably the single most important safety factor in polypectomy. It allows the assistant to stop snare closure before the wire withdraws too far into the tube, and there is danger of a smaller stalk being cut off by cheese-wiring mechanically without adequate electrocoagulation. It also warns if the stalk is larger than apparent or head tissue has become entrapped (Fig 7.4). Marking can, less conveniently, be performed *after* insertion by looking for the moment when the wire emerges from the snare catheter. Many snare handles have marker numbers molded-in or printed-on, but making a fresh physical mark is safer, because this proves that the point of wire closure has been exactly checked, and it is easier to see.

Other devices

• ***Hot biopsy forceps*** are occasionally used to destroy small polyps up to 3-4mm in diameter, and even for electrocoagulating telangiectases or angiodysplasia when argon plasma coagulation (APC) is unavailable.

• ***Injection needles*** are invaluable for saline or epinephrine (adrenaline) injection, whether for elevation of sessile polyps, to prevent or arrest bleeding, or to tattoo a polypectomy site.

• ***Dye-spray*** (***chromoscopy***) ***cannulas*** allow visualization or surface detail interpretation of small or flat polyps, and the margins of sessile polyps, although dye can (perhaps more easily) also be syringed in without a cannula.

• ***Clipping or nylon-loop placement devices*** have an occasional invaluable place, either to deal with postpolypectomy bleeding or to prevent it. The metal clips routinely available are too short-jawed to compress a thick stalk and a nylon loop is difficult to place over a large head. However either can be placed on the residual stalk when there is bleeding or increased risk of it, as in patients with a bleeding diathesis or on anticoagulants or similar medication. Ideally both a loop (EndoLoop®, Olympus) and a clipping device should be available, pre-primed in case of a sudden bleed. As they are relatively fiddly to assemble in a crisis, single-use clipping devices overcome this problem, a first gentle squeeze opening up the clip and a further (forcible) squeeze closing it.

• ***APC cannulas***, where used (see below), can be either forward- or side-firing, depending on the direction of gas flow outlet. Either variety works well in most circumstances, as the essential step is to produce a localized cloud of argon gas over the area to be electrocoagulated.

• ***Specialized accessories***, including "knives" (cutting wires), hooks, etc. are in evolution to make close-up endoscopic submucosal dissection (ESD) of large sessile lesions quicker and safer, but are outside the remit of most endoscopists.

• ***Specimen retrieval*** may be with the snare or one of the retrieval devices (such as the multi-wire "memory metal" Dormia basket

(Fig 7.5) or the nylon Roth net (Fig 7.6). Smaller polyps or portions up to 6–7 mm can be aspirated through the channel into a filtered suction trap (Fig 7.7) or, more cheaply, onto a gauze placed over the suction connector on the light guide plug at the end of the umbilical (Fig 7.8).

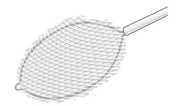

Fig 7.6 Nylon polyp retrieval net.

Principles of polyp electrosurgery

Electrosurgical or diathermy currents cause heat and coagulate local blood vessels. Coagulated tissue also becomes easier to transect with the snare wire, but this is of secondary importance. Heat is generated in tissue by the passage of electricity (electrons), the flow of which causes collisions between intracellular ions and release of heat energy in the process (Fig 7.9). The high-frequency or "radio-frequency" electric current used alternates in direction at up to a million times per second (10^6 cycles/s or 1 MHz) (Fig 7.10).

There is no "shock" or pain at such high frequencies because there is no time for muscle and nerve membrane depolarization before the current alternates again, and no muscle contraction

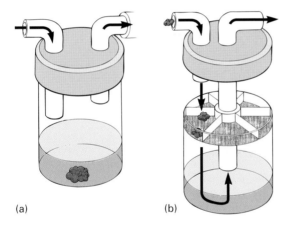

(a)   (b)

Fig 7.7 (a) An old-style mucus trap. (b) A filtered polyp suction trap.

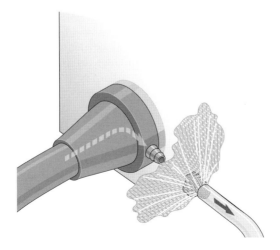

Fig 7.8 Gauze inserted over suction connector for polyp retrieval.

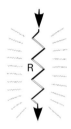

Fig 7.9 Heat is generated by electricity (electrons) passing through resistance (R)—in this case tissue.

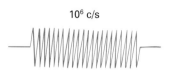

10^6 c/s

Fig 7.10 An electrosurgical current alternates 1,000,000 times per second, producing heat but no shock.

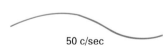

50 c/sec

Fig 7.11 A household current alternates 50–60 times per second, producing heat and shock.

or afferent nerve impulse. Electrosurgical current is therefore not felt by the patient and there is equally no danger to cardiac muscle. This is in contrast to low-frequency household currents, which shock because they alternate only 50–60 times per second (50 cycles/s) (Fig 7.11). At the low power used in polypectomy, even the unlikely possibility of a direct thermal burn to the skin of a patient or operator is surprising but trivial. Adhesive "patient plates" or return electrodes ensure good skin contact, and safety circuitry sounds a warning if proper connections have not been established. The only real danger from electrosurgical currents is their heating effect on the bowel wall at the site of electrocoagulation.

Modern cardiac pacemakers are unaffected at the relatively low power used for endoscopic electrosurgery. An additional safety factor is that the electrosurgical current passage between the polypectomy site in the abdomen and patient plate (usually on the thigh) is reasonably remote from the pacemaker. Implanted cardiac defibrillators, however, can be fired by electrosurgical currents and temporary deactivation of the defibrillator by a cardiac technician with full cardiac (ECG) monitoring of the patient is recommended at the time of polypectomy. If in doubt, consult the patient's cardiologist.

Coagulating and cutting currents

Cutting current has an uninterrupted (and so high-power) waveform of relatively low voltage spikes (Fig 7.12). The interrupted current flow excites the air molecules into a charged "ionic cloud," visible as high-temperature sparking that vaporizes the surface cell layer to steam. Because it is low voltage, however, cut current is less able to traverse desiccated tissue and to heat deeply.

Coagulating current has intermittent higher voltage spikes with intervening "off periods," which last for about 80% of the time (Fig 7.13). The higher voltage allows a deeper spread of current flow across desiccating tissue, whereas the off periods reduce (except at high power settings) the tendency for gas ionization, sparking, and local tissue destruction.

Blended current combines both waveforms (Fig 7.14), some units providing the ability to select blends with relatively greater "cut" than "coag" characteristics. The differences between the various makes of electrosurgical unit imply that the output characteristics

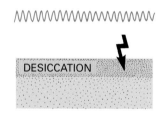

Fig 7.12 Cutting current—continuous (high-power) low-voltage pulses cannot pass desiccated tissue.

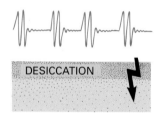

Fig 7.13 Coagulating current—intermittent high-voltage pulses can pass desiccated tissue.

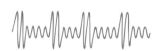

Fig 7.14 Blended current combines the characteristics of both cutting and coagulating currents.

are more complex than this brief summary suggests, some appearing to provide more effective hemostasis than others. When changing from one unit to another it is therefore essential to be cautious and to start with low-power settings. If possible, try out the unit on a small lesion or the periphery of a larger one, rather than entering the "big-time" unrehearsed and then regretting it.

"Auto-cut" current, produced by the circuitry of some "intelligent" electrosurgical units, will automatically adjust power output to match the resistance of the tissue being heated, the intention being to produce a predictable rate of transection. Although this may be a safety factor for some large sessile polyps in thin parts of the colon, we find that for routine polypectomies the hemostasis can be insufficient. The endoscopist also forfeits the ability to control the rate of severance and degree of local heating using the "feel" of snare closure (see below). We therefore prefer use of coagulating current (sometimes described as "soft coagulation" in such units).

Current density

Tissue heats because of its high electrical resistance, typically around 100 ohms, although resistance varies according to the particular tissue (fat conducts poorly and so heats little). Water loss (desiccation) during heating increases resistance, and the drying tissue is also mechanically harder to transect. If electric current is allowed to spread out and flow through a large area of tissue, the overall resistance and heating effect falls (Fig 7.15). To obtain effective electrocoagulation, the flow of current must be restricted through the smallest possible area of tissue; this is the principle of "current density" (Fig 7.16). This principle is basic to all forms of electrosurgery and explains why no noticeable heat is generated at the broad area of skin contact with the patient "return plate," whereas intense heat occurs in the closed snare loop (Fig 7.17). Even a relatively small area of contact between the buttock or thigh and patient plate is adequate. Extra moisture or electrode jelly is unnecessary at the power used for endoscopic polypectomy.

The essential in polypectomy is to heat-coagulate the core of the polyp stalk or base, with its plexus of arteries and veins, *before* transection. Closing the snare loop both stops the blood flow ("coaptation") and concentrates the current to flow through and heat-coagulate the core (Fig 7.18). Tightness of the loop is crucial, as the area through which the current is concentrated (current density) decreases as the square of snare closure (πr^2), thus causing a square law relationship between snare closure and increasing current density. The heat produced increases as the square of current density, so heating increases as the *cube* of snare closure (i.e. a slight increase of snare closure on a polyp stalk greatly increases the heat produced). Conversely, the fact that the closed snare loop is the narrowest part of the stalk means that the base of the stalk and the bowel wall should scarcely heat at all, which explains the rarity of bowel perforations during or after stalked polypectomy. Contact pressure between snare wire and polyp surface and thickness of snare wire (thinner wire, greater heating)

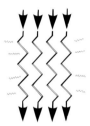

Fig 7.15 Current flows more easily through larger areas of tissue resistance and so produces little heat.

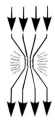

Fig 7.16 Current density results from constricting tissue and greatly increases heating.

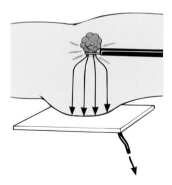

Fig 7.17 Heating occurs at the closed snare but not at the plate.

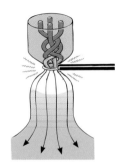

Fig 7.18 The whole plexus of stalk vessels must be electrocoagulated before section.

are additional factors, with a square law relationship between contact area and heat produced.

Coagulation increases proportionately to increase in power setting on the unit dial (Fig 7.19) and *increases directly as time passes* (ignoring complicating features such as heat dissipation) (Fig 7.20).

Closure of the snare loop is the most important variable, because of the cubed increase of heat production as the snare closes (Fig 7.21). If the snare is too loose it will hardly heat the tissue at all; if too tight it will heat the tissue too fast. The soft stalk of a small polyp should, therefore, coagulate rapidly. A larger stalk, being less compressible, requires a slightly higher power setting and more time before visible tissue coagulation occurs. Visually it can be difficult to be absolutely sure of the diameter and consistency of the stalk, as the view may be poor and the wide-angle lens distortion can be confusing. The "feel" of the stalk may also be inaccurate, especially with snares having a thin and compressible plastic sheath, which can result in the snare handle being "closed" when the stalk is actually inadequately narrowed (Fig 7.22). It is to allow for this "crumpling" under pressure that a check for loop closure 15 mm within the sheath is so important before snaring a large polyp with a new snare type. Similarly, it is to allow time to react to what is happening that the recommendation is to perform polypectomy using coagulating current only, and at a low power setting (corresponding to only 15–25 W). Only occasionally should it be necessary to increase the power if no visible coagulation has occurred; extra time will usually do the job. The "auto-cut" setting of some electrosurgical units adjusts output automatically for appropriate heating during snaring.

"Slow cook" is the essential principle of polypectomy, so as to electrocoagulate an adequate length of stalk tissue before section. There should be visible whitening as the protein denatures, with swelling (or even steam) as stalk tissue boils. Remember that some tissue necrosis may extend beyond the zone of obvious electrocoagulation whitening (which is why mucosal ulceration and secondary bleeds occur after "hot biopsy"). However, if all the water boils off, electrons will no longer flow through the desiccated tissue of a polyp stalk and the wire may have to be pulled through mechanically—in principle a somewhat risky thing to do, because

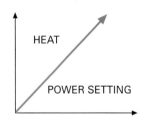

Fig 7.19 Heat produced is directly proportional to power . . .

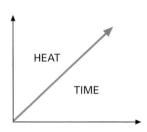

Fig 7.20 . . . and directly proportional to time . . .

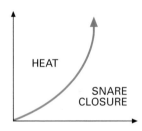

Fig 7.21 . . . but *increases* as the *cube* of snare closure.

thick-walled vessels are usually the last part to sever. Inevitably it takes a little time at the safer lower current settings to heat the tissue. If this takes more than 30–40 seconds, the risk of heat dissipation at a distance (and damage to the bowel wall) increases and it may be more realistic to increase the power setting to speed things up. The maximum power setting used should be equivalent to no more than 30–50 W.

Thick stalks (1 cm or more in diameter) are more difficult to coagulate, with a risk of inadequate central vascular electrocoagulation, particularly if the stalk is firm and relatively noncompressible and the plexus of vessels within it are large and thick-walled. A higher power setting may be needed to start electrocoagulation peripherally and tight snaring may also be needed to start electrocoagulation. This combination can have unfortunate effect that, as the snare starts to transect and close down through the stalk, the heat produced increases very dramatically. This results in electrocutting of the central core, precisely the part that needs slow and controlled coagulation. Additional factors such as current leakage from "contralateral" contact points may complicate things further, as discussed later.

If no visible coagulation is occurring in a large polyp stalk check:
- *whether the circuitry and connections are correct*
- *whether the snare is properly assembled and fully closed*
- *whether the stalk has been correctly snared* or the head trapped out of sight (see Fig 7.4)
- *if the stalk is very thick*, and if so consider epinephrine injection (see Fig 7.23) and have nylon loop or clip ready
- *whether the snare loop can be repositioned higher up the stalk* where it is narrower.

If there is any fear of complications or the operator is inexperienced, this may be the moment to disengage the snare and leave the procedure to someone else (see below for how to disengage a "stuck" snare).

Polypectomy

Stalked polyps

Even an expert can have difficulty snaring some polyps. A beginner, unskilled in handling the colonoscope, can miss seeing them or get inadequate views of the polyp, resulting in unsafe or incomplete snaring.

The following steps and points should help guarantee safe and effective polypectomy.

1 *Check and mark the snare*. An overenthusiastic but inexperienced assistant can cheese-wire through the polyp stalk before adequate electrocoagulation by closing the snare handle too forcibly. This is particularly likely if the snare wire is thin or the polyp stalk is small. The mark on the snare handle indicates the point at which the tip of the snare loop has closed down to the end of the outer sheath. This can be done visually beforehand or when the snare is already within the colon (see Fig 7.3). When a thick stalk

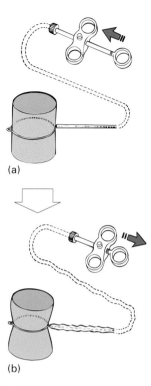

(a)

(b)

Fig 7.22 When snaring a thick stalk (a) the plastic sheath may crumple before closure is adequate (b).

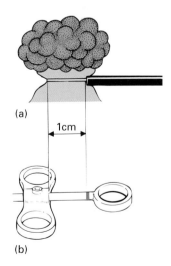

(a)

1cm

(b)

Fig 7.23 (a) Thick stalks can bleed—think of pre-injection. (b) The distance to the closure mark indicates the stalk size.

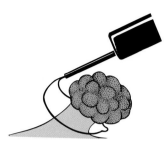

Fig 7.24 Backward snaring is sometimes useful.

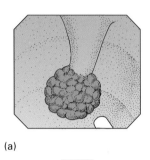

(a)

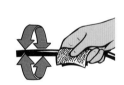

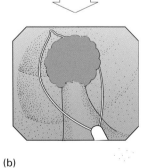

(b)

Fig 7.25 (a) Bad position for snare placement? (b) Rotate the instrument to get a better working position and view.

is snared the mark gives a useful approximate measure of its size and a warning that there may be problems (Fig 7.23b).

2 *Get to know the electrosurgical unit.* When first using an electro-surgical unit, start with the lowest dial setting and use initial bursts of 2–3 seconds at each increased setting. Discover the lowest dial setting (usually 2.5–3) that causes visible controlled electrocoagulation in the smallest stalk.

3 *Develop a standard routine for polypectomy* and always follow it. Check the connections, plate position and the electrosurgical unit setting before each polypectomy. Make sure that the foot pedal is in a convenient position, preferably where it can be felt with the foot without having to look down to search for it at the crucial moment after the polyp is grasped. A polyp can suddenly shift if the patient moves or coughs.

4 *Use the closed snare outer sheath to assess the base or stalk mobility* of larger polyps. Visual assessment of the stalk size can be difficult due to the distorting effect of the wide-angle endoscope lens. Comparing the stalk size to the 2-mm width of the protruded plastic snare sheath and pushing it around to assess length and mobility can be invaluable, warning that extra power and/or longer time will be needed for transection.

5 *Open the snare loop within the instrument channel* when snaring small or average-sized polyps. This avoids the need to manipulate the snare handle when the loop emerges from the endoscope. Lassoing the polyp head efficiently takes practice. It is usually best to have the loop fully open, and then to maneuver only with the instrument controls or shaft, so that the snare loop is placed over the polyp head almost entirely by manipulation of the endoscope. It may help to open the snare in the colon beyond the polyp, and then to pull the colonoscope slowly back until the polyp head comes into the field of view and into the open loop. Alternatively, the loop can be pushed backward over a difficult polyp head (Fig 7.24), or placed to one side or other of the polyp head and then swung over it by appropriate movements of the instrument.

6 *Optimize the view and position of the polyp* before becoming committed, especially if the polypectomy looks as though it may be awkward, which is often only apparent after trying to place the loop over the polyp head (Fig 7.25a). A change of patient position can improve the view of the stalk. Rotate the colonoscope shaft to exit the snare in the ideal position, at the bottom right of the field of view, so that the view is not lost during polypectomy (Fig 7.25b).

7 *Snare the polyp and push the snare sheath against the stalk* (the "push" technique), which ensures that closing the loop will tighten it exactly at the same point. If the sheath is not pushed against the stalk, loop closure by the assistant will tend to move or even pull the wire off the polyp (Fig 7.26) unless the endoscopist simultaneously advances the sheath (the "pull" technique). If there is any doubt that the snare is properly over the polyp head, try shaking the snare or opening and closing the loop repeatedly to help it slip down around the stalk. Vigorous angulation of the colonoscope tip in the relevant direction may help, even if this means losing the ideal view.

8 *Close the snare loop gently*, to the mark or by feel, until it is properly closed. Snare closure occurs ideally near the top of the stalk at its narrowest part, leaving a short segment of normal tissue to help pathological interpretation (Fig 7.27). Initial snare closure should be gentle; the loop may be in the wrong place and if the wire has cut into polyp tissue it may be difficult to release and reposition. With longer stalks, especially if there is any suspicion of malignancy, it may be possible and desirable to snare lower down the stalk so as to increase the chance of resecting all invasive tissue.

9 *If the snare loop is stuck in the wrong position*, or if it becomes apparent that the polyp cannot be safely transected, releasing the snare is made easier by lifting up the loop over the polyp head and pushing forcibly inward, with the whole colonoscope if necessary (Fig 7.28). If the loop is ever completely trapped in a polyp, a second, small-diameter instrument (gastroscope or pediatric colonoscope) can be inserted alongside the first scope and the biopsy forceps used to coax the wire free. Remember that it is always possible (depending on type) either to dismantle the snare or to sacrifice it by cutting it outside the patient with wire cutters, withdrawing the colonoscope and leaving the loop *in situ*. Either the polyp head will fall off or another attempt can be made with a new snare (or, if necessary, a different endoscopist). It is never necessary to be "committed" to a polypectomy just because it has been started.

10 *Electrocoagulate using a low-power coagulating current* (15 W or dial setting 2.5–3, but perhaps one setting higher for larger polyps) with the snare loop kept *gently* closed to "neck" the tissue and create favorable circumstances for electrocoagulation. Apply the current continuously for 5–10 seconds at a time, watching for visible swelling or whitening. Once the stalk or base below the snare is visibly coagulating, squeeze the handle more tightly while continuing electrocoagulation, and transection will start.

11 *Watch where the polyp head falls*, or time may be wasted looking for it. If it is lost, look for any fluid, which indicates the dependent side of the colon where the severed polyp head is likely to have fallen. If no fluid is visible, squirt in some water with a syringe and watch where it flows. If the water simply refluxes back over the lens, the polyp will also be distal to the instrument tip and the endoscope needs to be withdrawn to find the specimen (Video 7.1).

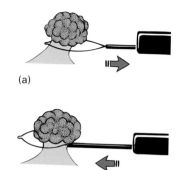

Fig 7.26 (a) To avoid the snare pulling off during closure (b) push the loop against the stalk before closing.

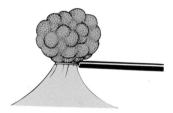

Fig 7.27 Snare at the narrowest part of the stalk.

Small polyps—snare, "cold snare," or "hot biopsy"?

Tiny polyps can sometimes be just as awkward to snare as larger ones, and difficult to retrieve even using the filtered suction trap. There has therefore been a tendency for some endoscopists to ignore small polyps or to describe them as "hyperplastic," wrongly inferring that small polyps have no neoplastic potential. On biopsy, 70% of such small polyps prove to be adenomas, and only around 20% of those in the colon (as opposed to the rectum) are hyperplastic. Small polyps in the colon should therefore be snared or destroyed on sight. The best method of doing this is a matter of debate (Video 7.2).

Forceps destruction can be appropriate for miniscule (1–1.5mm) polyps.

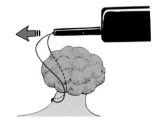

Fig 7.28 To disengage a trapped snare, push it upstream over the polyp head.

Mini-snares (9–10mm loop size) are convenient for snaring most small (2–7mm) polyps, opening predictably within the close-up view required. However, by coordinating carefully with the assistant when opening and closing the loop, a standard (25mm) or larger loop can be used if a mini-snare is not available.

Snaring small polyps accurately can be technically demanding. Some skill is needed to lassoo the tiny lesion at its base, and then to locate and aspirate the severed specimen for histology.

Conventional snare electrocoagulation presents no problem, except that electrosurgical transection can occur too fast, before sufficient (visible) coagulation has occurred. It may therefore be best for the endoscopist to take control of the snare handle in order to ensure controlled loop closure.

"Cold snaring," with no electrocoagulation, relies on physical traumatization of vessels during transection to cause local vasoconstriction and accelerated coagulation. Providing that the polyp has been accurately snared, no care is needed in snare closure and the procedure is rapid and easy, immediate bleeding being surprisingly uncommon (and easily controlled by epinephrine injection if necessary), and the significant hazard of delayed postpolypectomy bleeding (secondary hemorrhage) virtually eliminated.

Aspiration into a suction trap (see Fig 7.7) is a convenient way of managing polyps up to 5–7mm in diameter. A gauze in the suction line is cheaper and just as effective for single polyps, the endoscopist being made aware that the specimen has arrived in the gauze by the silence of the blocked suction line (see Fig 7.8). Larger specimens usually impact at the opening of the instrument channel unless fragmented by the snare or in the suction process.

"Hot biopsy"

Electrocoagulation with insulated forceps can be a quick and effective way of destroying the smallest (1–4mm) polyps with simultaneous representative histology (Fig 7.29a). However, over the years their use occasionally results in surprisingly large (1–2 unit transfusion) secondary bleeds occurring 1–12 days afterwards, probably when unintentionally deep-tissue heating and necrosis damages a local arteriole. Hot biopsy has therefore largely been abandoned in favor of cold-snaring small polyps.

Hot biopsy forceps are only different from conventional diagnostic forceps in having a plastic insulation outer sheath and an electrical connector for the cable to the electrosurgical unit, via a patient plate, just as for polypectomy. The same low-power "coag" setting (15–25W or equivalent) is used as for snaring a small polyp. The specimen taken (often only 10–20% of the whole polyp) is protected from current flow within the forceps jaws, and so is unheated (unless by thermal conduction resulting from over-lengthy current application). By contrast, provided that the technique is properly performed, within 1–2 seconds there is intense local heating of the polyp tissue and the feeding blood supply, resulting in surprisingly dramatic but superficial ulceration—which heals over the next 2 weeks.

Safe hot biopsy depends on localizing the heating effect by careful attention to details of technique.

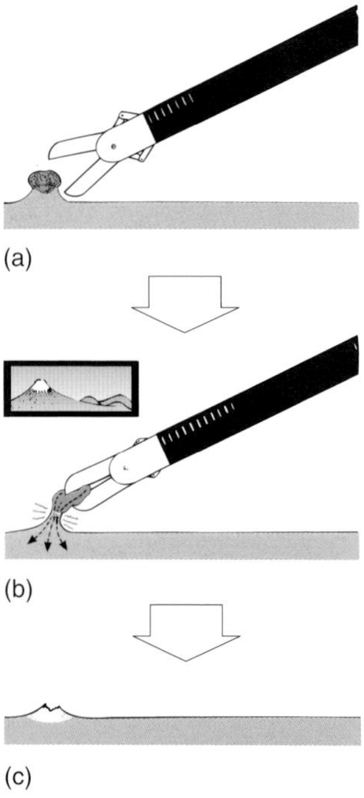

(a)

(b)

(c)

Fig 7.29 Hot biopsy forceps grasp the small polyp (a) and pull up and coagulate until there is "snow on Mount Fuji" (b), then pull off the biopsy sample, leaving the coagulated polyp base (c).

1 *Select only a suitably small polyp*—and be prepared to abandon hot biopsy and change to (mini-)snaring if the grasped polyp proves to be bigger than expected.

2 *Grasp only the apex of the small polyp* in the jaws of the hot biopsy forceps (Fig 7.29b), deliberately *not* forcing the jaws into the colon surface below, as would be normal in taking a mucosal biopsy.

3 *"Tent up" the polyp onto a "pseudo-pedicle"* (like a small mountain) by colonoscope angulation or by withdrawing the forceps slightly. This elevation is made possible because of the loose stroma of submucosa over the underlying colon wall (analogous to that of the skin over the back of the hand). It is hazardous in the thin proximal colon, where many endoscopists feel that use of hot biopsy is contraindicated (and great care must be taken).

4 *Ensure that the insulating plastic of the forceps is visible*, so that the metal parts of the jaws do not contact the endoscope.

5 *Apply coagulating current for a maximum of 2–3 seconds*. Because the pseudo-pedicle is the narrowest part, local current density should result in almost immediate heating and electrocoagulation. The extent of coagulation is visible as whitening, but this should ideally spread only halfway down the "mountain"—the "Mount Fuji effect" (Fig 7.29c). Further spread is unnecessary, as even normal-looking tissue is heated and will subsequently become necrotic.

6 *Pull off the biopsy* in the knowledge that, even if some of the head is left uncoagulated, the basal tissue and blood vessels will have been destroyed and it will slough off.

Polyps of 4mm in diameter or more are not suitable for hot biopsy. Either the base will be broader than the area of contact of the forceps (so only a small burn will result at the surface of the polyp) or, more dangerously, the current will fan out from the point of contact of the hot biopsy forceps (Fig 7.30) (heating tissue at a distance, invisibly causing necrosis). Coagulating for too long or attempting to destroy over-large polyps with the hot biopsy technique therefore risks causing a deep ulcer with the chance of delayed hemorrhage or even of full-thickness heating and perforation (both risks especially great in the proximal colon). So, if a polyp proves to be too large for rapid and localized visible electro-coagulation, *stop*, take the biopsy, and remove the rest of the tissue by conventional snare polypectomy.

Problem polyps
Sessile polyps

It is difficult to achieve "current density" for localized heating when snaring a sessile or broad-based polyp. This is why removal of large sessile polyps (Fig 7.31a) or broad-stalked polyps presents problems for the endoscopist and why piecemeal removal can be the safer option (see also ESD and "en bloc" removal, below). For such lesions "auto-cut" electrosurgical units may be an advance, because they provide the high power needed to start transection but reduce it rapidly to safer levels thereafter. Fortunately, many so-called "sessile" polyps up to 10–15 mm in diameter are simply "semi-pedunculated" or, if "broad-based," can be pulled up by the snare onto an adequate and compressible pseudo-stalk. Alternatively

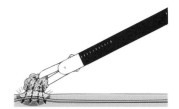

Fig 7.30 Hot biopsy—dangerous heating if the polyp is too big or doesn't tent up.

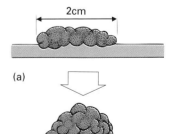

(a)

(b)

Fig 7.31 (a) Sessile polyps can be risky to snare in one portion . . . (b) . . . because "tenting" results.

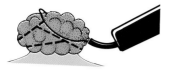

Fig 7.32 Piecemeal removal is safer (although less satisfactory for the pathologist).

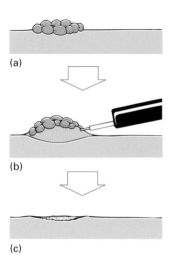

(a)

(b)

(c)

Fig 7.33 (a) A small sessile polyp . . . (b) . . . is elevated by submucosal saline injection . . . (c) . . . and snared off in one piece.

submucosal injection can be used to elevate the polyp tissue before snaring (see below).

Move the closed snare to and fro as a measure of safety having snared all or part of a sessile polyp; if the mucosa moves, but not the bowel wall, there is no danger. If the colon moves with the snare, the full thickness of the wall has been "tented" dangerously (Fig 7.31b) and the snare should be repositioned to take only a smaller part. If the base of a protuberant polyp is over 1.5 cm in diameter, with no stalk, the safe course is to take the head piecemeal in a number of bits (Fig 7.32). Each bit can be cut through with no risk of full-thickness burns and little risk of bleeding, as the vessels of the head are much smaller than those in the stalk. With the submucosal injection technique described below, however, it may be possible to remove flat sessile polyps up to 1.5–2 cm in diameter in a single specimen, and much larger ones piecemeal.

Endoscopic Mucosal Resection—"injection polypectomy"

Submucosal saline injection elevates sessile polyps for easier removal, a technique common in proctology and originally described for colonoscopic use in 1973 (Video 7.3). Injection has become a frequent routine, initially with the intention of obtaining small sessile polyps (flat adenomas) as a single histopathological specimen (Fig 7.33). "Injection polypectomy" or endoscopic mucosal resection (EMR) can also be invaluable for the removal of much larger polyps, having the double advantage of creating a bloodless (when epinephrine is used) plane for transection and a "safety cushion" of engorged submucosal stroma that protects the bowel wall from heat damage. Injection can be with normal saline (0.9%) or 1 : 10,000 epinephrine in 0.9% saline (1/200,000 epinephrine concentration), but this absorbs in 2–3 minutes, so snaring needs to be reasonably quick. To make the injected bleb last longer, a hypertonic solution can be injected (2 N saline, 20% dextrose, or hyaluronic acid have all been used, with or without epinephrine). Some experts add a few drops of methylene blue when making up the solution, the blue showing up the extent of the submucosal bleb and helping to outline the edge of a sessile lesion. With a 10 mL syringe attached, a sclerotherapy needle (25G) is aimed tangentially to the mucosal surface adjacent to the polyp, then the injection made by one of two approaches:

• *the "push technique"* (preferred option) requires the assistant to start injecting *before* the needle tip jabs in and penetrates about 1–2 mm under the mucosal surface;

• *the "pull technique"* has the needle first jabbed in under the mucosal surface or through the polyp tissue, only then starting injection as the needle is slowly withdrawn.

A relatively slow, low-pressure injection gives time, if necessary, to note that a submucosal bleb is forming. The "plane of separation" in the submucosa for successful injection is surprisingly superficial and the tendency is to inject too deep, although there is no hazard involved should the needle or solution pass into the peritoneum (or the peritoneal cavity). An injection of 1–3 mL should be enough to raise the submucosa below a small polyp for immediate snaring, but 20–30 mL may be needed for larger polyps and up to 100 mL for giant hemi-circumferential lesions.

Make the first injection proximal to a large sessile polyp, so that the raised bleb of tissue does not obscure the view. Make each subsequent injection into the edge of the preceding bleb (Fig 7.34) or inject directly through the polyp surface (providing the polyp is thin enough for the needle to reach the submucosa below).

Failure of injection to elevate a sessile polyp ("non-lifting sign") *suggests malignancy*, the lesion being fixed by invasion into deeper layers. If non-lifting occurs, take no risks in attempting total removal but wait for histology and consider assessment by endoscopic ultrasound or other form of scanning. Surgery is likely to be necessary. Always remember to tattoo the site to help localization.

Large sessile polyps—piecemeal polypectomy

Even very large sessile polyps can usually be removed endoscopically, but this may require special skills and should be a matter of expert opinion and clinical judgment (Video 7.4). It has been suggested that sessile polyps occupying more than 50% of the colon circumference, or involving two haustral folds, are too big for safe endoscopic removal, but opinion is changing as technical skills and accessories evolve. The endoscopic approach is the obvious one in a patient who is a bad operative risk and is prepared to accept repeated endoscopy. If colonoscopy is technically difficult, it may be better to consider laparoscopy.

At the first endoscopic session attempt complete removal (even if *piecemeal)*, because scarring will make subsequent attempts at submucosal injection and removal less likely to succeed. Injection is a significant help in safe debulking, but the main requirements are endoscopic dexterity, patience, and sufficient time. Piecemeal removal of a very large polyp can take an hour or so. Any basal remnants are easily and safely destroyed with APC (Fig 7.35). Before finishing, a submucosal tattoo is left adjacent, to facilitate follow-up.

A pediatric scope can be used in retroversion to pre-inject or snare the proximal part of a polyp if it proves to be difficult to see or target. Standard polypectomy snares sometimes slip off the moist and domed pre-injected area, whereas a stiffer thin monofilament snare can be effective for cutting into the polyp or the bleb beneath it (bleeding is not a significant risk in sessile polyps). A "needle-knife" has been used by some to pre-cut around the injected and raised polyp margin, allowing the snare to grip it better. A spike-tipped snare can fix the tip of the snare into the mucosal surface at an appropriate point, making opening and control of the loop easier. The tip of a standard snare can be similarly anchored by (very brief) electrocoagulation of the tip, fixing it into mucosa.

Pain during sessile polypectomy, unless due to overinsufflation, is a warning that full-thickness heating of the bowel wall is occurring, activating peritoneal pain receptors. Fortunately pain is felt before there is any risk of serious damage—another reason for avoiding heavy sedation or anesthesia. If pain occurs and deflation

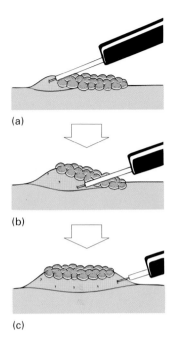

(a)

(b)

(c)

Fig 7.34 (a) First inject *proximally* to a larger sessile polyp . . . (b) . . . then around the periphery . . . (c) . . . to elevate it completely before snaring.

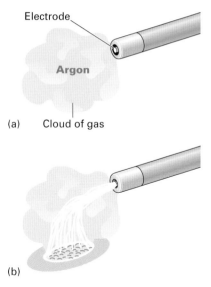

Fig 7.35 (a) Argon plasma coagulation (APC) catheter with internal wire electrode emits argon gas cloud. (b) Activating electrosurgical unit ionizes gas, conducting current to tissue (and patient plate).

does *not* stop it (it is easy to be overenthusiastic with the air button when trying to keep a good view during a problematic polypectomy), the procedure should be abandoned until another session at least 3 weeks later, when healing should have occurred and the area can be properly assessed.

Large polyps and endoscopic submucosal dissection

Consider flexible endoscopic removal of large sessile polyps in the rectum. Sessile polyps up to 12 cm from the anal verge are extraperitoneal (below the peritoneal reflection), so relatively safe from perforation. They can be removed by local proctological techniques, which often produce a single large specimen for optimum histology, rather than the chaos of fragments resulting from endoscopic piecemeal snaring, but the surgical view is poor. *Transanal microsurgery* (TEMS) under anesthesia potentially allows anal dilation and two-handed approach for injection, scissor-excision or full-thickness removal if malignancy is suspected, but the technique is cumbersome and not widely available. The technique of *endoscopic submucosal dissection* (ESD) is an attractive alternative endoscopic approach for large sessile lesions, particularly in the rectum and in skilled hands. The technique is adapted from Japanese approaches to endoscopic treatment of early gastric cancer, which can be removed en bloc using a combination of submucosal injection and "free-hand" dissection using a variety of electrosurgical knives. The technique is slow, however, and technically demanding, so should be left to experts with appropriate experience.

As already stated, a failed initial endoscopic attempt to remove such rectal polyps forms scar tissue, which then greatly hinders any subsequent attempt at submucosal excision, so the endoscopist's decision to refer to an appropriate expert (whether for EMR, ESD, or local transanal surgery) should be made on the basis of visual assessment alone, without either biopsy or attempted snare removal if this seems likely to fail.

Submucosal injection for EMR or ESD in the rectum should be with 1:200,000 epinephrine solution (compared with 1:10,000 in the rest of the colon) because there is risk of communication to the systemic circulation and serious cardiac dysrhythmia.

Smaller rectal polyps close to the anal canal can be snared in retroversion and after local anesthetic injection (typically with 3-5cc of 2% lignocaine solution, but without epinephrine for safety reasons). The distal 3–5 cm of the rectal ampulla is otherwise difficult to visualize properly and is also richly supplied with sensory nerves, a heat burn causing the same pain as it would on exterior skin. If the polyp is very small and quick to snare, "cold-snaring" may be the best approach.

Avoid the trap of snaring internal hemorrhoids (or localized varices) in the distal rectum, which can result in highly impressive bleeding.

Large stalked polyps

The "large" size of a polyp is sometimes an illusion because the visual judgment of size is made relative to the diameter of the colon lumen. Proximal colon and cecal polyps thus tend to be *larger* than they look at first sight. In the narrowed lumen of diverticular disease, polyps that appear large may prove on snaring to be significantly *smaller*.

In snaring a large stalk, extra electrocoagulation is needed to minimize the increased chance of bleeding from the relatively large plexus of stalk vessels, and extra care (and time) should be taken to optimize things before starting.

1 *Check that an epinephrine-filled injection cannula can be rapidly available* in case of bleeding, and probably a clipping device and nylon EndoLoop® as well.

2 *Palpate and move the stalk* around using the closed snare to judge its diameter, length, and mobility.

3 *Get the best view possible*; if necessary rotate the endoscope or change patient position (Figs 7.25 and 7.36).

4 *Place the snare optimally on the narrowest part of the stalk* to ensure maximal current density.

5 *Consider "pre-snaring" lower down the stalk* in order to extend the zone of electrocoagulation. Squeeze the snare *gently* for this preliminary stalk heating, so that transection does not occur and the snare is easy to release and replace higher up the stalk for conventional polypectomy.

6 *Electrocoagulate the stalk* for longer than usual, until visible swelling and whitening indicate that it is safe to start transection.

7 *Consider using a higher than usual current setting*, especially if, in the process of transection, the core desiccates and the snare will not make the final cut. Resist the urge to "pull through" the snare. The thickest arteries are the last to sever, so it is safer to raise the current setting further and let heat help to make the cut.

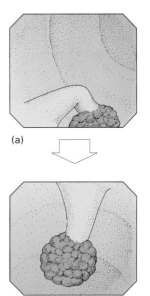

(a)

(b)

Fig 7.36 (a) Bad view of a polyp? (b) Change the patient's position to let gravity help.

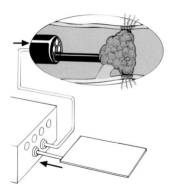

Fig 7.37 "Leak" current can result in contralateral burns.

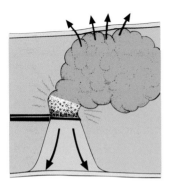

Fig 7.38 A large area of contact reduces the risk of contralateral burn, but also reduces current flow and heat coagulation in the lower stalk.

In snaring large-stalked polyps, complications, especially bleeding, need to be anticipated (and so often avoided). Large polyps inevitably have larger, thicker-walled, and more numerous feeding vessels. By employing a careful "slow cook" polypectomy technique, the precautionary methods described below and the crisis-control (or prevention) accessories, we have experienced no serious immediate hemorrhage after polypectomy for many years. Delayed bleeds, however, do continue to happen unpredictably, maximally in the first 24–48 hours, but for up to 12–14 days on occasion.

Contralateral burns are essentially a "non-problem." During snaring of a large stalked polyp, the head will flop about, inevitably touching the bowel wall in several places. "Leak" currents flow at each point of contact, which results in inefficient heating of the stalk (Fig 7.37) and the possibility of a contralateral burn—often out of the field of view. The burn hazard is mainly theoretical and the possibility can be avoided by moving the snared polyp head around during coagulation, which ensures that no one point gets all the heat. Alternatively make sure that the area of contact between the head and the opposite wall is large, so that resistance is low and local heating insignificant.

During a difficult polypectomy try to keep a view of the snared stalk, especially if only part of the polyp can be seen, and ensure that adequate visible coagulation occurs *below* the snare loop before transection. (If leak currents do flow up the stalk to a contact point at the head, electrocoagulation can occur primarily *above* the snare (Fig 7.38) and bleeding could result from inadequately coagulated vessels in the lower part of the stalk.)

If there is any doubt about stalk electrocoagulation when the polyp head has severed and if the stalk remnant shows too little visible electrocoagulation whitening, or visible vessels at the center, it may be wise to "post-snare" lower down, squeezing the stalk gently and electrocoagulating further (without transection) before reopening and removing the loop.

Stalk pre-injection with epinephrine before snaring may make immediate bleeding less likely (Fig 7.39a). Epinephrine (1–10 mL 1 : 10,000 dilution in 0.9–1.8% (1 N or 2 N) saline) is injected at one or more sites into the base of the polyp and causes visible blanching from vessel contraction within a minute or so. The endoscopist sees blanching and swelling of the stalk, and finally mauve coloration

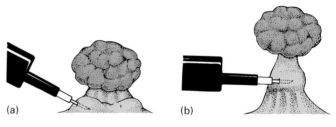

(a)   (b)

Fig 7.39 (a) Inject broad-stalked polyps with epinephrine before snaring to avoid bleeding. (b) For long-stalked polyps with a risk of bleeding inject sclerosant and epinephrine.

of the ischemic head. Transection through the upper part of the stalk or above the injected area can then be made with greater confidence.

Nylon loops or metal clipping devices are particularly relevant to large-stalked polyps or, in patients on anticoagulants or aspirin, as a way of strangulating the remaining stalk. The most certain method for larger stalks is the nylon self-retaining EndoLoop® (Fig 7.40). The loop is usually placed on the stalk remnant *after* polypectomy, because the floppy loop is difficult to maneuver over a polyp head of 2 cm or more. For smaller stalks, one or more metal clips can be placed easily before or after snaring. Clips are particularly useful in controlling local bleeding after sessile polypectomy when there is no stalk on which to close a loop (Video 7.5).

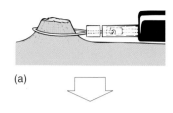

(a)

Recovery of polypectomy specimens

Extraction of large polyps (3 cm or more) through the anal sphincters can be difficult. The polyp will often fragment if excessive traction is needed on the snare or retrieval grasper, although a multi-wire Dormia basket or Roth polyp-retrieval net should avoid this if it can be coaxed over all or most of the polyp specimen. Once at the anus ask the patient to help extraction by bearing down "as if to pass wind," which reflexly relaxes the sphincters. At the same time gentle traction is applied to produce the polyp (cover the perineal area to avoid explosive surprises!).

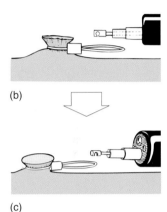

(b)

(c)

If withdrawal fails in the left lateral position, the patient can be asked to squat on the floor or sit on a commode seat, which is more physiological and (with traction maintained on the retrieval device) rapid expulsion of the polyp invariably results. A large rigid anoscope and tissue-grasping or sponge-holding forceps can alternatively be used, pulling out the polyp and instrument together.

Fig 7.40 (a) A nylon self-retaining loop can be placed over a large stalk . . . (b) . . . and its self-retaining cuff tightened; (c) . . . and the loop unhooked leaving the stalk strangulated.

Multiple polyp recovery

Ninety percent of adenoma patients have only one or two polyps, and it is uncommon to find more than five. Some multiple polyps (hyperplastic, Peutz–Jeghers, juvenile, lymphoid, lipomatous, or inflammatory) are non-neoplastic, so that it may sometimes be preferable to await results of standard biopsies or representative polypectomies before undertaking heroic numbers of polypectomies, which are probably more risky than the lesions themselves.

If a patient has six or more obvious adenomas, fortunately a rare occurrence, it is essential to examine the whole colon before snaring and to be certain that multiple smaller polyps are not present (with the possibility of a diagnosis of familial adenomatous polyposis (FAP)). Looking for tiny reflective nodules in the "light reflex" of the transparent mucosal surface shows up polyps down to 1 mm in diameter that are invisible to direct vision, but very obvious on dye spray. Melanosis coli also shows up tiny nonpigmented polyps or lymphoid follicles very well. Take representative biopsies for certainty of diagnosis, either way.

Dye spray ("*chromoscopy*") enhances the view of fine detail, almost to dissecting microscope level. The principle is to spray the surface with dye (0.1–0.4% indigo carmine solution), which shows up any small polyps down to under 0.5 mm in size, as pale islands on a blue background. Dye can be applied using a dye-spray catheter, usually during withdrawal of the scope. An easier method is to use 5 mL of dye in an air-filled 20–30 mL syringe inserted into the rubber biopsy valve of the scope. This allows a short segment of colon to be dyed in only a few seconds without using a catheter. Silicone-emulsion anti-bubble solution can be added to the dye to avoid small bubbles, which can look confusingly like tiny polyps. Histology of any polyp seen is essential for certainty because lymphoid follicles can resemble adenomas to the untutored eye (although usually dimpled or "umbilicated" at their centers).

Digital chromoendoscopy: Narrow band imaging (NBI) and Fuji Intelligent ChromoEndoscopy (FICE) use different methods to narrow the bandwidth of white light, picking out different parts of the visual spectrum to enhance the visualisation of different tissues. NBI uses optical filters to enhance the central spectrum, picking out the increased microvascular density and enabling adenomas to become more visible against the surrounding mucosa. FICE is based on spectral estimation technology and uses a post-endoscopy processing system. Both are activated by the push of a button on enabled scopes, which has clear advantages over the use of dye-spray. Digital chromoendoscopy may have utility in high-risk groups where spotting even diminutive adenomas is important for risk stratification, for example hereditary non-polyposis colorectal cancer (HNPCC) patients.

Retrieval of multiple polyps for histology is a matter of compromise in order to avoid needing to reinsert the colonoscope repeatedly. In practice retrieval can be facilitated by use of accessories such as the Roth polyp-retrieval net which can, with care and some skill, retrieve up to three to five moderately large polyps at a time, whereas only one or two polyps can be picked up in the polypectomy snare. Any smaller polyps are either destroyed by hot biopsy or snared and then aspirated into a filtered polyp suction trap or into a gauze placed in the suction line (see Fig 7.7). A "wash-out" technique is a rarely needed compromise after the snare removal of large numbers of non-neoplastic polyps (Peutz–Jeghers syndrome, juvenile or inflammatory polyposis). On first presentation of some such patients, as many as 60–100 polyps may need removal, although their histology is of secondary interest, as there is little or no malignant potential. The multiple snared polyps are first retrieved to the descending or sigmoid colon, the colonoscope is then passed to the splenic flexure and 500 mL of warm tapwater is syringe-injected through the instrument channel. The proximal colon is air-insufflated until the patient feels some distension and, just before the colonoscope is withdrawn from the anus, a disposable or phosphate enema can be injected through the endoscope. This ensures evacuation and passage of most of the polyps or polyp fragments into a commode within a few minutes.

Inflammatory polyps of 1 cm or larger should be removed, as sporadic adenomas can occur in colitis patients. Most post-inflammatory polyps, sometimes called pseudo-polyps, appear as small, shiny, worm-like tags of healthy and non-neoplastic tissue after the healing of previous severe colitis of any kind. They can be ignored or, if in doubt, a few biopsies can be taken to confirm their trivial nature. Larger post-inflammatory polyps have a tendency to bleed, and there may be difficulty in distinguishing them from adenomas, as they can be composed of granulation tissue or disorganized tissue remarkably similar to that of a hamartomatous (juvenile) polyp. These larger polyps can bleed surprisingly after snaring, partly because they tend to have soft bases that "cheese-wire" through too quickly compared with the more muscular pedicle of other polyps, but also because they may be very vascular. Any broad-based or sessile polyp, and especially any raised plaque occurring after longstanding ulcerative or Crohn's colitis must be treated with suspicion, as it may represent a so-called "DALM" (dysplasia-associated lesion or mass), the most visible part of a "field change" of high-grade dysplasia. With such dubious lesions, take mucosal biopsies around the base before snaring to discount this possibility.

Malignant polyps

Malignancy may be suspected if a polyp is irregular, ulcerated (0–2c Paris classification), firm to palpation, thick-stalked, or fails to lift with submucosal injection (non-lifting sign). Close inspection of pit pattern with dye (Kudo classification type V) or absent vascular pattern with NBI (NICE type 3) should alert the endoscopist to the possibility of invasive malignancy. If doubt remains regarding the suitability of endoscopic resection, endoscopic ultrasound (EUS) can be employed, although many endoscopists take a pragmatic approach by assessing the lifting characteristics and aim to resect if lifting is adequate. If a pedunculated "polyp cancer" is possible, it is important to be certain that transection is made low down the stalk (to allow the pathologist proper assessment) and to ensure that any invasion within the stalk has been removed, without risking perforation. The pathologist should report, on the basis of multiple vertical cross sections, whether or not the polyp has been completely removed, but the endoscopist's opinion as to whether removal has been complete is also important and should be recorded. If necessary an early repeat examination can be made, preferably within 2 weeks while there is visible healing ulceration to indicate the polypectomy site (and allow biopsy and tattooing). Because of the possibility of malignancy, each polyp is ideally retrieved and identified separately on an anatomical "colon map" in a biopsy book kept available in each endoscopy room. It is inadequate to say that a polyp was removed at "70 cm from the anus" because this might equally represent the mid-sigmoid colon or cecum.

Tattooing should mark the site of any suspicious or partially removed polyp, whether for follow-up or possible surgery. A solution of suspended sterile carbon particles (commercially available in a syringe as SPOT®) is injected intramucosally (Fig 7.41). A volume of 1 mL adjacent to the polypectomy site may be sufficient for endoscopic follow-up, but if surgery or laparoscopy is a possibility, making multiple tattoos on several sides of the colon should ensure easy visibility at surgery regardless of which way the bowel

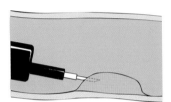

Fig 7.41 A 1 mL India ink tattoo marks a polypectomy site permanently.

is lying (tattoos are not necessary or recommended for rectal lesions, as surgical tissue planes may be disrupted by fibrosis induced by the ink). The problem of ink leakage and "black out" of the endoscopic view can be avoided by first injecting a small saline bleb (or blebs) submucosally, and then changing syringes so that the 1–2 mL tattoo aliquot enters the bleb. The carbon particles remain in the submucosa for many years (probably for life), easily visible to the endoscopist as a blue-gray stain. Sterilized India ink is an alternative to suspended carbon particles, although does not have a formal licence for medical use, and a syringe-mounted bacterial filter may be required (Video 7.6).

Adequate removal of a malignant polyp is a recurrent problem, especially if the histopathologist's report of malignancy comes as a surprise to the endoscopist. Nonspecific features of large size, induration, or irregular surface may arouse suspicion, but the macroscopic appearance of a malignant polyp can be unremarkable. The clinician or endoscopist is then faced with a dilemma but, happily, one that can usually be resolved in favor of conservatism (rather than surgery), certainly for pedunculated polyps. If the cancer is histologically "well" or "moderately well" differentiated, with a margin of 1 mm or more between the limit of invasion and the transection line, and assuming that endoscopic removal also appeared complete, surgery is *not* recommended. The likelihood of there being residual local tumor or resectable lymph node involvement under these circumstances is extremely small (ignoring the even more remote, but ever present, possibility of unresectable distant metastases), whereas the 1% mortality of surgery in older patients is immediate.

Surgery is indicated for a malignant polyp **when**:
* *the polyp is sessile*;
* *invasion extends histologically within 1 mm of the resection line*;
* *the carcinoma is poorly differentiated* (*anaplastic*), and so more likely to metastasize.

Under these circumstances the likelihood of involved lymph nodes is significant and most would favor operation, *unless* the patient is considered to be a poor surgical risk. Clinical judgment is involved, balancing risks and clinical factors in the interests of long-term survival. Review of the histological slides is essential and a second opinion from a specialist histopathologist may be indicated. The opinion of the patient or the patient's family should be sought and may also swing the decision. If there is any doubt, it may be difficult not to operate in a young patient, mainly for emotional reasons and for "absoloute safety." In older patients the decision is not so obvious; very few patients have been found at operation to have locally involved resectable lymph nodes or residual tumor even when the histology appears "unfavorable," but some patients found to have *no* residual cancer have died as a result of the (unnecessary) surgery. Operation does not, in any case, guarantee freedom from residual cancer; there have been reports of subsequent death from distant (micro-) metastases in spite of normal operative findings by the surgeon and histopathologist.

Complomplications

Bleeding is the most frequent complication of polypectomy—usually "delayed" 1–14 days after polypectomy, but occasionally "immediate" after transection. Bleeding (whether immediate or delayed) should complicate less than 1% of small polypectomies, although reported rates for larger (>3 cm) sessile polyps requiring piecemeal polypectomy are between 7 and 14%. Hemorrhage from large polyp stalks has become rare, as endoscopists have appreciated the need for maximum "slow-cook" stalk electrocoagulation, and the usefulness of epinephrine injection and nylon-loop or clip strangulation.

Immediate bleeding is usually a slow ooze but can be an arteriolar spurt of frightening proportions, as viewed endoscopically. Every possible attempt should be made to stop an arterial bleed immediately, as any delay can result in the view being lost or in clot formation. Infusing large volumes of water prevents clotting if blood obscures the view of the bleeding point. Clots are impossible to aspirate, but moving the patient to improve visualisation (for example to the right side to visualize the distal colon), localization of the polypectomy site and endoscopic therapy should be possible. Quickly re-snare the remaining stalk, inject epinephrine (up to 5–10 mL of 1 : 10,000 solution) submucosally into or adjacent to the stalk remnant or use APC electrocoagulation. If the stalk has been re-snared, simple strangulation alone (taping the snare handle closed for 10–15 min) is usually sufficient without further electrocoagulation. If bleeding recurs on releasing the snare, further electrocoagulation, use of APC or endo-clips will stop it. Alternatively, re-grasp the stalk, apply squeeze pressure, and then use injection through a second instrument (pediatric colonoscope or gastroscope) passed up alongside the first. In the unlikely event that arterial bleeding persists in spite of all efforts, the most elegant solution is to perform selective arterial catheterization and embolization or infusion of vasopressin (success has been reported using vasopressin or somatostatin by intravenous infusion alone). A surgical team must be alerted and adequate supplies of blood ensured.

Secondary (delayed) hemorrhage can occur for up to 12–14 days, particularly after snaring of larger polyps or hot biopsy of overlarge (over 5 mm) polyps. Delayed bleeds may be more frequent or more persistent in patients on antiplatelet agents, which normally should be stopped 7–10 days beforehand if multiple or large polypectomies are predicted. Persistent or secondary hemorrhage in the left colon will be indicated by repeated calls to stool and the passage of fresh clots, whereas in the right colon the rate of bleeding is more difficult to assess because of the long delay before altered blood is expelled.

All patients who have had polypectomy should know of the possibility of delayed bleeding, partly for reassurance if minor bleeding occurs. They should have the relevant telephone numbers and be told to report to hospital for admission should blood loss be persistent or substantial. Delayed hemorrhage normally stops spontaneously but transfusion (and perhaps repeat colonoscopy) is occasionally required and the possibility of angiographic control should not be forgotten.

The "postpolypectomy syndrome," with fever, pain and peritonism, represents "closed perforation" with full-thickness heat damage to the bowel wall. It is an occasional sequel to a difficult polypectomy, especially after piecemeal removal of a large sessile polyp in the proximal colon. Localized abdominal pain and fever persist for 12–24 hours following polypectomy, but without free gas on x-ray or signs of generalized peritonitis. The inflammatory reaction of the peritoneum should result in adherence by local structures (typically covering by omentum or small bowel), so it is a self-limiting event. Conservative management with bed rest and systemic antibiotics is indicated, but surgical consultation is wise if the symptoms and signs do not abate rapidly.

Frank perforation is fortunately rare. Management may often be conservative, but this depends on the area of the polyp base. A small polyp removed by snare or hot biopsy in a well-prepared bowel is obviously "lower risk," whereas signs of perforation after a larger or sessile lesion in a poorly prepared colon mandate surgery. A surgeon should always be alerted; if in doubt, it is safest to operate—laparoscopic oversewing or clipping of the affected area is the preferred option (Video 7.7).

Safety

Any polypectomy is potentially hazardous, so adherence to all possible safety measures is essential. Assuming that the correct equipment is available, it must be carefully handled and maintained. If polypectomy is not proceeding according to plan, check the electrosurgical settings, connections, and patient plate circuitry before anything else.

The greatest single safety factor lies in a strict routine, regularly repeated for each polypectomy, because human error is much more likely than equipment failure. A military-type approach has much to commend it, with any request from the endoscopist being repeated out loud by the assistant so that each knows what the other is doing. The assistant and the endoscopist must check on each other to watch that all is in order during the procedure, having checked the equipment (including marking the snare handle at the point of closure) beforehand.

Good bowel preparation is essential to give a good view and a dry field in which to work. If bowel preparation is poor, as during flexible sigmoidoscopy, use carbon dioxide instead of air to prevent the possibility of explosive combinations of oxygen (from inflated air) with methane (from bacterial metabolism of protein residues) or hydrogen (from bacterial fermentation of carbohydrates). Alternatively, take great care to insufflate and then aspirate repeatedly to dilute any gas present. In a well-prepared bowel there is no explosion hazard and air can be safely used.

Patient medications may be of importance. To minimize the risk of delayed hemorrhage, clopidogrel or other medications affecting platelet adhesion should ideally be withdrawn for 10 days before (to allow a new generation of "sticky" platelets to form) and for 7–14 days after the procedure. Recent data supports current recommendations that polypectomy is safe for patients on aspirin or nonsteroidal anti-inflammatory drugs (NSAIDs). Many endoscopists will proceed with polypectomy even if the patient is found unexpectedly to be on antiplatelet medication, providing the patient will have easy access to medical care and there is no social or travel contraindication. Scrupulously careful technique and due warning to the patient about the possibility of delayed bleeding are indicated.

Only a very experienced operator should undertake polypectomy in a patient remaining on anticoagulants. The patient should be warned of the possible need for immediate repeat endoscopy should delayed bleeding occur, since spontaneous cessation is less likely. Very careful precautions should be taken, including saline injection before polypectomy, and safety loops or clips perhaps placed afterwards. Often, with the approval of the relevant clinician, anticoagulants can be stopped for the 10–12-day period needed to cover the procedure and the likelihood of immediate or delayed bleeding after polypectomy. Some favor admission of the patient to hospital and transfer to heparin for the immediate post-polypectomy period, but the major risk of (delayed) bleeding comes later, often after discharge from hospital.

Other therapeutic procedures

Balloon dilation
Balloon dilation of short strictures and anastomoses is easy with "through-the-scope" (TTS) balloons, especially those with an internal guidewire. TTS balloons now furl tightly enough to pass through small-diameter instruments (although a standard 3.7 mm channel gives better feel and control). The balloon is silicone-spray lubricated before insertion. The instrument shaft and tip is straightened as much as practicable to minimize insertion force and avoid kinking. To achieve this it may be necessary to withdraw the scope a little and pass back to the stricture once the balloon is in position. The integral guidewire makes insertion through angulated or fixed strictured areas substantially easier, but dexterity, handling skill, and imagination are often needed to coax the balloon into position.

Balloons of at least 18 mm diameter give the best long-term results and those that are 5 cm long are easiest to "dumb-bell" within the stricture, staying put rather than slipping in or out during distension. Balloons must be fluid-distended, using either water or dilute contrast material, because air is too compressible. A pressure-gun and manometer are used, because it is impossible by hand to reach and sustain the recommended distension pressures—typically around 5 bar or 80 psi (pounds per square inch)—for the 2 minutes needed to dilate effectively, especially as the balloon plastic slowly stretches a little. The gun also allows the pressure control needed for "controlled radial expansion" balloons, which give the endoscopist a reasonably precise idea of the dilation diameter achieved.

Dilation is hazardous and how far to dilate is a matter of judgment. The overall perforation rate for stricture dilation in different series ranges between 4% and 10%, so properly informed consent must be obtained beforehand, and the patient should appreciate that there is a small but significant risk of ending up in the operating theater. Very scarred, ulcerated, or angulated strictures are more likely to split under dilation (perhaps dilate to 12–15 mm initially and repeat to a larger diameter on another occasion). Postsurgical anastomotic strictures are safer and easier to dilate, especially if "straight on." Metallic stents (see below) may have a place in managing the most obstinate and fibrous stenoses. However, the typically web-like fibrous bands that can occur at some anastomotic strictures are susceptible to "needle-knife" incision before large-diameter balloon dilation, with excellent results.

Tube placement

Deflation and tube placement is important in ileus or "pseudo-obstruction" (Ogilvie syndrome), where endoscopic deflation avoids the need for surgery. Unless a drainage tube is left, ideally inserted into the proximal colon, simple colonic deflation tends to be short-lived in effect. Different methods are available.

A purpose-designed colon drainage set is available for TTS insertion, or components of an endoscopic retrograde cholangiopancreatography (ERCP) stent set can be used, cutting holes in the pusher tube before inserting it over the guidewire, leaving the tube behind and withdrawing the guidewire. Frequent irrigation of the tube is likely to be needed because of its small diameter.

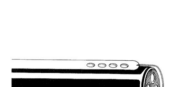

Fig 7.42 A deflation tube can be carried up alongside the colonoscope.

A "piggy-back" method carries up a larger drainage tube alongside the scope, a loop attached to the leading end of the tube being grasped by forceps (Fig 7.42). A variation avoids using the forceps and allows better suction during the procedure (the colon may be unprepared and foul): a thin loop of cotton thread at the end of the tube is held by a loop of strong monofilament nylon passed through the suction channel; once in the proximal colon a sharp tug on the nylon loop breaks the cotton thread and the tube is free. The drainage tube is attached to a suction pump or drainage bag. The tendency of the deflation tube to be ejected by colonic movement can be prevented by stiffening it with a guidewire (Savary–Gilliard or similar steel-wire type), silicone-lubricated for insertion.

Volvulus and intussusception

The colonoscope can be used to deflate a *sigmoid volvulus*, effectively acting as a steerable flatus tube, so that the deflated loop can de-rotate passively. A deflation tube (as above) can be inserted through the instrumentation channel. However, after the tube or endoscope tip has been passed gently into or through the twisted segment, deflation alone is usually sufficient for the torsion to reverse spontaneously, so endoscopic manipulation is usually unnecessary. Only if the segment appears blue-black and gangrenous from ischemia is surgery indicated, because of the high risk of perforation.

Intussusception is easy to diagnose but usually impossible to reduce colonoscopically because not enough inward push can be transmitted around the looped colon to the ileo-cecal area (where this rare event most commonly occurs). Identifying and removing any causative factor, such as a large polyp or lipoma, should help prevent recurrence.

Angiodysplasia and hemangiomas

In treating angiodysplasia it is best to err on the side of applying too little heat. Even minor whitening and edema will progress to produce remarkable local ulceration within 24 hours. It is easy enough to repeat the examination a few weeks later to check results, but difficult to justify perforation from overaggression during the first procedure. As angiodysplasias occur mainly in the thin-walled proximal colon, great care should be taken with whichever modality is used—preferably APC because of its ease, efficacy, and relative safety. If this is unavailable, any other form of electrocoagulation (mono- or bipolar), heater probe, or laser, can be carefully applied. The judicious use of hot biopsy forceps is particularly effective with smaller lesions, which can be grasped, the mucosa tented up, and selectively heated. It is unnecessary to take a biopsy, and the jaws are simply reopened after minimal visible coagulation (Video 7.8). In larger angiodysplasias that have an obvious central "feeding vessel" it is preferable to create a ring of local heating points around the periphery, followed by one or more applications near the center, rather than to apply excessive heat in one area alone and risk bleeding or perforation (Fig 7.43).

Larger angiodysplasias should be tackled last, and the most dependent ones treated first, because they may bleed and cause others to be missed. The object of coagulation is to damage the superficial part of the vascular lesion (which extends also into the submucosa), coagulating the vessels nearest the surface that are most liable to trauma, but also causing regrowth of normal mucosa over the top of the remaining vessels. If several angiodysplasias are present it can be difficult to be certain which has been the source of bleeding. Surface ulceration is a rare but obvious stigma of recent bleeding; a small bright-red lesion, well perfused from below, is more suspect than a larger but superficial, spidery and pinkish one. Mucosal trauma or spots of blood are easy to mistake for angiodysplasia; if in doubt irrigate the surface or traumatize the "lesion" to see if it bleeds. This is better than overdiagnosing and risking a complication unnecessarily.

Hemangiomas invariably have snake-like, very tortuous, vessels. There is great variation in colon vessel pattern, and a corresponding tendency to overdiagnose vascular abnormality. Endoscopic therapy is in any case ineffective in generalized hemangiomas, so examination is simply to exclude other lesions and document the appearance. Only the rare polypoid protuberances of childhood "cavernous hemangiomas" (blue rubber bleb nevus syndrome) are endoscopically treatable, whether by APC or sclerotherapy (they can occur throughout the gastrointestinal tract, as well as in the skin and elsewhere).

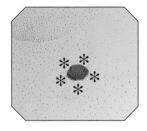

Fig 7.43 Point coagulation around an angiodysplasia before heating the center.

Tumor destruction and palliation

Debulking and vaporization of inoperable or obstructing tumor tissue is possible, using any combination of snaring, APC, or laser photocoagulation. Multiple injections of 100% ethanol using a sclerotherapy needle have also been used, the procedure being repeated every day or two until the desired clearance is achieved. In the rectum a urological resectoscope loop has been used, as for transurethral prostatectomy, either under glycine solution or in air.

Insertion of self-expanding metal stents has largely replaced such heroics. The stents used are similar to esophageal stents but, partly because tumor ingrowth is slow and easily managed but stent migration is a problem, colonic stents are uncoated and their nitinol "memory metal" construction is deliberately made to be immovable (so also unremovable). Insertion of colonic stents is normally a combined endoscopic–fluoroscopic procedure. Ideally the endoscopist inserts the scope proximal to the tumor, passing the guidewire and allowing precise localization of the upper and lower margins either by means of metal clips or radiological skin markers. Occasionally formal dilation may be needed, but usually there is slow spontaneous (and much safer) dilation of the stent over the next 24 hours. If an endoscope will not pass the strictured area, a hydrophilic "J-wire" can be inserted under direct vision, contrast injected down its catheter and the rest of the procedure and stent insertion managed under fluoroscopic control. The endoscopist checks for satisfactory location and expansion of the distal end of the stent.

Further readings

General sources

Waye JD, Rex DK, Williams CB. *Colonoscopy* (2nd Edition). Oxford: Blackwell Publishing Ltd, 2009, 816 pp. Extensively referenced multi-author textbook covering all aspects.

Waye JD, Aisenberg J, Rubin PH. *Practical Colonoscopy*. Oxford: John Wiley & Sons, Ltd. 2013, 199pp. A good overall account of the "nuts and bolts" of colonoscopy, but particularly strong on polypectomy.

Polypectomy techniques

Canard JM, Vedrenne B. Clinical application of argon plasma coagulation in gastrointestinal endoscopy: has the time come to replace the laser? *Endoscopy* 2001; **33**: 353–7.

Ellis KK, Fennerty MB. Marking and identifying colon lesions. Tattoos, clips, and radiology in imaging the colon. *Gastrointest Endosc Clin North Am* 1997; **7**: 401–11.

Ferrara F, Luigiano C, Ghersi S et al. Efficacy, safety and outcomes of "inject and cut" endoscopic mucosal resection for large sessile and flat colorectal polyps. *Digestion* 2010; **82**: 213–20.

Heldwein W, Dollhopf M, Rösch T *et al.* Munich Gastroenterology Group. The Munich Polypectomy Study (MUPS): prospective analysis of complications and risk factors in 4000 colonic snare polypectomies. *Endoscopy* 2005; **37**: 1116–22.

Repici A, Hassan C, Vitetta E *et al.* Safety of cold polypectomy for <10 mm polyps at colonoscopy: a prospective multicenter study. *Endoscopy* **2012**; **44**: 27–31.

Repici A, Hassan C, Vitetta E *et al*. Safety of cold polypectomy for <10 mm polyps at colonoscopy: a prospective multicenter study. *Endoscopy* **2012**; **44**: 27–31.

Tanaka S, Oka S, Chayama K, Kawashima K. Knack and practical technique of colonoscopic treatment focused on endoscopic mucosal resection using snare. *Dig Endosc* 2009; **21** Suppl 1: S38–42.

Tappero G, Gaia E, DeGiuli P *et al*. Cold snare excision of small colorectal polyps. *Gastrointest Endosc* 1992; **38**: 310–13.

Wadas DD, Sanowski RA. Complications of the hot-biopsy forceps technique. *Gastrointest Endosc* 1987; **33**: 32–7.

Endoscopic aspects of polyps and cancer

Cappell MS, Abdullah M. Management of gastrointestinal bleeding induced by gastrointestinal endoscopy. *Gastroenterol Clin North Am* 2000; **29**: 125–7.

Clements RH, Jordan LM, Webb WA. Critical decisions in the management of endoscopic perforations of the colon. *Am Surg* 2000; **66**: 91–3.

Haggitt RC, Glotzbach RE, Soffer EE, Wruble LD. Prognostic factors in colorectal carcinomas arising in adenomas: implications for lesions removed by endoscopic polypectomy. *Gastroenterology* 1985; **89**: 328–36.

Lieberman D. Colorectal cancer screening: practice guidelines. *Dig Dis* 2012; **30** Suppl 2: 34–8.

Rex DK, Bond JH, Feld AD. Medical-legal risks of incident cancers after clearing colonoscopy. *Am J Gastroenterol* 2001; **96**: 952–7.

Toyonaga T, Man-i M, Chinzei R *et al*. Endoscopic treatment for early stage colorectal tumors: the comparison between EMR with small incision, simplified ESD, and ESD using the standard flush knife and the ball tipped flush knife. *Acta Chir Iugosl* 2010; **57**: 41–6.

Ueno H, Mochizuki H, Hashiguchi Y *et al*. Risk factors for an adverse outcome in early invasive colorectal carcinoma. *Gastroenterology* 2004; **127**: 385–94.

Chapter video clips

Video 7.1 Stalked polyps

Video 7.2 Small polyps

Video 7.3 Polypectomy: EMR

Video 7.4 Piecemeal polypectomy

Video 7.5 Endoloop

Video 7.6 Tattoo

Video 7.7 Postpolypectomy bleed with therapy

Video 7.8 APC for angiodysplasia and polyp eradication

CHAPTER 8

Resources and Links

Websites

There is a huge amount of valuable material on the Internet, posted largely by the main endoscopy societies around the world. These include many thoughtful guidelines for practice. A full list of national societies is available from Organisation Mondiale de Endoscopy Digestive (OMED) at www.omed.org and links to all published guidelines can be found at www.gastrohep.com.

The main (Western) society resources are:

American College of Gastroenterology (ACG). Available online at www.acg.gi.org

American Gastroenterological Association (AGA). Available online at www.gastro.org

American Society for Gastrointestinal Endoscopy (ASGE). Available online at www.asge.org

British Society of Gastroenterology (BSG). Available online at www.bsg.org.uk

European Society for Digestive Endoscopy (ESDE). Available online at www.esge.com

Society for American Endoscoping Surgeons (SAGES). Available online at www.sages.org

Endoscopy books

Classen M, Lightdale CJ, Tytgat GNJ. *Gastroenterological Endoscopy.* Stuttgart, New York: Thieme, 2002, 777 pp. *A comprehensive multi-author review.*

DiMarino AJ, Benjamin SB. *Gastrointestinal Disease: an Endoscopic Approach.* Boston: Blackwell Science, 1997, 1161 pp. *A comprehensive two-volume textbook focusing on the clinical practice of gastrointestinal endoscopy.*

Modlin IM. *A Brief History of Endoscopy.* Milano: Multimed, 2000. *Not so brief—a fascinating and detailed historical review, including the history of endoscopic societies.*

Schiller KFR, Cockel R, Hunt RH, Warren BF. *Atlas of Gastrointestinal Endoscopy and Related Pathology* (2nd edn). Oxford: Blackwell Science, 2002. *Detailed text and multiple images, incorporating pathology.*

Shepherd M, Mason J, Swan CJ. *Practical Endoscopy.* Chapman Hall Medical, 1997. *An excellent introduction aimed primarily at nurses and endoscopy assistants.*

Sivak M (ed.) *Gastroenterologic Endoscopy* (2nd edn). Philadelphia: WB Saunders, 2000. *The biggest textbook to date (120 contributing authors, 1611 pages).*

Sivak MV, latterly Lightdale CJ (series ed.) *Gastrointestinal Endoscopy Clinics of North America.* Philadelphia: WB Saunders.

Waye JD, Rex DK, Williams CB. *Colonoscopy. Principles and Practice.* Oxford: Blackwell Publishing, 2003.

Journals with major endoscopy/clinical focus

American Journal of Gastroenterology. Official Journal of the American College of Gastroenterology.

Digestive Endoscopy. Official Journal of the Japan Gastroenterological Endoscopy Society.

Endoscopy. Official journal of the European Society of Gastrointestinal Endoscopy, and 20 affiliated national societies.

Gastrointestinal Endoscopy. The official journal of the American Society for Gastrointestinal Endoscopy.

Gut. Official journal of the British Society of Gastroenterology.

Surgical Endoscopy. Official journal of the Society of American Gastro¬intestinal Endoscopic Surgeons and European Association for Endoscopic surgery.

Cotton and Williams' Practical Gastrointestinal Endoscopy: The Fundamentals, Seventh Edition.
Adam Haycock, Jonathan Cohen, Brian P Saunders, Peter B Cotton, and Christopher B Williams.
© 2014 John Wiley & Sons, Ltd. Published 2014 by John Wiley & Sons, Ltd.
Companion Website: www.wiley.com/go/cottonwilliams/practicalgastroenterology

Epilogue: The Future? Comments from the Senior Authors

Old folks like to look back, as Peter did recently in writing his memoirs "The tunnel at the end of the light; my endoscopy journey in six decades" (available online at www.peterbcotton.com). It is more challenging to look forwards, but it is always fun to try.

The start of our careers coincided with the birth of modern endoscopy and it has been a privilege to see and to nurture its progressive march into the heart of gastroenterological practice. As we fade into the sunset it is tempting to assume that the best is over. That is doubtless wrong. It is impossible to anticipate the paradigm shifts that could occur with undreamed of advances in technology, but less difficult to make some predictions by extrapolating from current trends. Here are a few ideas:

Intelligent endoscopes

Modern lives are much enhanced by computer chips. Our cars know where they are, how far they have been, how to get places, how much further they can go before refueling and servicing, even the pressure in the tires or when dangerously close to other objects. Experimental cars are now cruising the open road without needing drivers. Thirty years ago one of us had a prototype self-steering colonoscope (model use only) with a joystick allowing control of its servomotor steering. Future endoscopes should gain some of these electronic functions. We look forward to scopes being able to steer themselves or to stay automatically in the center of the lumen, know where they are and have been, to recognize what they see and report it, and to give advice when needed—quite apart from keeping track of faults and repairs and key quality metrics. Maybe they will be able to decide whether a particular endoscopist is competent, and to design any necessary remediation programs. And, while the engineers are busy realizing our dream endoscopes, they may wish to focus also on improving the ergonomics.

Colonoscopy—boon or bubble?

Most gastroenterologists nowadays are consumed by performing colonoscopy, largely for screening purposes. While this is clearly beneficial (as well as remunerative), it has distorted practice and compromises the consultative role for which they were trained. Currently, doctors do the procedures and leave much of the talking to patients to "mid-level providers," i.e. nurse practitioners and physician assistants. In our view, the reverse would be preferable, and will likely occur for several reasons. Although colonoscopy will doubtless become technically easier, no one can claim that it is either cheap or noninvasive, as screening methodology is supposed to be. Ideally colonoscopy should become a second-tier, mainly therapeutic, procedure for patients selected by other simpler methods. These could perhaps include capsule colonoscopy or advanced CT colonography, but, ideally, screening will be by genetic testing or cell sampling using genetic, proteomic, or other biomarkers. We can expect pharmacological or immunological methods for preventing and/or treating polyps.

In the interim, colonoscopy is already widely practiced (independently) by trained nurses in the UK. This will happen eventually in the USA and elsewhere as demand increases but procedure reimbursement continues to fall. Of course, highly trained colonoscopists will still be needed for complex cases.

Advanced therapeutics, cooperation, and multidisciplinary working

Endoscopists took over a huge part of digestive "turf" from surgeons in the 1970s and 80s when the main

Cotton and Williams' Practical Gastrointestinal Endoscopy: The Fundamentals, Seventh Edition.
Adam Haycock, Jonathan Cohen, Brian P Saunders, Peter B Cotton, and Christopher B Williams.
© 2014 John Wiley & Sons, Ltd. Published 2014 by John Wiley & Sons, Ltd.
Companion Website: www.wiley.com/go/cottonwilliams/practicalgastroenterology

therapeutic procedures were developed and disseminated. Techniques have been refined since that time, but new frontiers are still being explored. Endoscopic mucosal resection (EMR) has become mainstream, and pioneers are going deeper. Working in the submucosa allows removal of neoplastic lesions and also peroral endoscopic myotomy (POEM) for achalasia. The last decade has seen attempts at exploration of an entirely new frontier for endoscopy, the abdominal cavity. Many natural orifice transluminal endoscopic surgery (NOTES) procedures have been performed in animals, and some in humans. It is to the credit of endoscopic and surgical leaders that these extraordinary developments are being explored ethically and in collaboration. The special individual talents of advanced endoscopists and laparoscopic surgeons are needed.

It is a truism that obesity is a major, and growing, problem worldwide. Bariatric surgery procedures are becoming popular, at least in Western countries. Attempts to mimic surgical approaches through the mouth are far advanced, and it is safe to say that this will be a fertile field for interventional endoscopists in the future.

The traditional separation between surgery and medicine, most evident in prestigious teaching institutions and privileged countries, was understandable in the Middle Ages but is now outdated and unhelpful. Our belief has always been that endoscopy is a tool of digestive specialists, not a specialty in itself, which led in 1980 to the merger of the British Society for Digestive Endoscopy with the Gastroenterology Society. There are many organizations relevant to endoscopy in the USA (AGA, ASGE, ACG, SAGES, and SGNA, among others) and thinly veiled hostilities and prejudices exist in many other countries. Despite intermittent attempts to work together on key issues, such fragmentation diminishes efficacy, authority, and influence—particularly in the all-important areas of training and performance standards. Cross-fertilization and cooperative interdisciplinary working should become the norm.

Quality and teaching

The recent focus on quality in endoscopy will grow progressively, propelled by patient empowerment, the drive for efficiency, and payment by outcomes rather than procedures. Is it too much to expect a day when endoscopy is performed only by those properly trained to do it, with outcome data fully available to the public? One of us has argued repeatedly in the USA (and without apparent impact) for some form of certification of endoscopists, at least for advanced procedures such as endoscopic retrograde cholangiopancreatography (ERCP). In this respect the "driving test" established for screening colonoscopists in the UK is a good precedent. "Train the trainers" courses are in vogue around the world, which helps to ensure that good habits are ingrained from the start, replacing or supplementing the traditional approach of slavish apprenticeship to a (supposed) master.

Our hopes for fully realistic and effective computer simulation have so far proved unachievable. This has principally been because of the requirements for stupendously fast processing to reproduce the interactions between the flexible scope and its accessories within the changing dynamics of the gastrointestinal tract, all necessarily at modest cost because of limited teaching budgets. Fortunately, multi-user video-gaming initiatives are driving phenomenal advances in processing speed and high-quality computer graphics, so we remain optimistic.

One of the consequences of aging is the expectation of requiring more personal medical interventions. We trust that anyone offering us an endoscopy in the future will be on top of their game (and hope that this little book may have helped in the process).

Peter Cotton & Christopher Williams,
March 2013

Index

Cotton and Williams' Practical Gastrointestinal Endoscopy: The Fundamentals, Seventh Edition.
Adam Haycock, Jonathan Cohen, Brian P Saunders, Peter B Cotton, and Christopher B Williams.
© 2014 John Wiley & Sons, Ltd. Published 2014 by John Wiley & Sons, Ltd.
Companion Website: www.wiley.com/go/cottonwilliams/practicalgastroenterology